S0-ARK-073

YOUR PERSONAL VITAMIN PROFILE

Your Personal Vitamin Profile

A Medical Scientist Shows You How to Chart Your Individual Vitamin and Mineral Formula

Dr. Michael Colgan

WILLIAM MORROW AND COMPANY, INC.
New York *1982*

THIS BOOK IS NOT intended for the treatment of illness but rather for its prevention. If you are ill, seek the services of a physician competently trained in nutrition. Advice given herein is for people in normal health who wish to remain that way. Any application of the advice herein is at the reader's discretion and sole risk. Readers are urged to consult the medical references given to decide for themselves the adequacy of the conclusions reached in this book.

Library of Congress Cataloging in Publication Data

Colgan, Michael.
Your personal vitamin profile.

Bibliography: p.
Includes index.
1. Vitamins in human nutrition. I. Title.
QP771.C64 1982 613.2′8 82-12560
ISBN: 0-688-01505-0
ISBN: 0-688-01506-9 (pbk.)

Printed in the United States of America

4 5 6 7 8 9 10

BOOK DESIGN BY BERNARD SCHLEIFER

To my dearest Lesley,
and to Bo,
a wonderful, courageous lady

FOREWORD

READER, count yourself lucky. The book you hold in your hands is the key to what you most desire. Who does not wish for extra years of healthful life, for themselves and their loved ones? Who does not wish for improved physical and mental abilities, for freedom from cancer, heart disease, arthritis, stroke and senility? This book provides the information you need. The choice is up to you.

During the last decade or two, scientists have learned as much about the causes of good health and disease as had been learned in the previous centuries. Recently the information has reached the "critical mass" stage, but until now no one has assembled it in a manner that is easily understood and easily applied. Dr. Michael Colgan has now systematically and brilliantly compiled—in his laboratory, in his clinics, and in the scientific libraries—the last bits of research you need to move yourself into a new era of vitality.

Perhaps that sounds familiar, maybe too familiar, and you are skeptical. I don't blame you for being skeptical. Every day, it seems, we have been told about a new wonder drug, a medical miracle of some sort that will prevent or cure cancer and heart disease, arthritis and a host of other maladies. All too often these miracles of modern medicine have proven to be disastrous. They usually don't work, and they usually bring about side effects that are as bad as or worse than the problems they were supposed to correct. To those still awed by the men and women in the white coats and stethoscopes, Dr. Colgan's discussion of the multiple failures of the traditional medical approach to health and disease will prove enlightening, if not downright startling. I totally agree with Dr. Colgan's advice: "If you need medical help, seek a nutritionally oriented doctor." The old recommendation "ask your doctor" is no longer valid. It never was.

Dr. Colgan resoundingly rejects the current medical approach to degenerative disease, except where the illness has reached crisis proportions for the individual. He recognizes that only by following nature's plan, rather than fighting it, can good health and optimum functioning be achieved. Nature's plan for man and animal is and always has been good nutrition, sufficient exercise and avoidance of toxic substances. Now, however, science has discovered how to isolate and synthesize the fifty or so nutrients that our bodies require, so we may take as much as we need to live and function at the *optimum* level, not just at the marginal or *survival* level. This book is your guide to that knowledge.

You will find much of the information Dr. Colgan provides to be both surprising and convincing. It takes an unusual individual to break sharply with the past and yet maintain scientific credibility. Dr. Colgan *is* an unusual individual. Dr. Colgan started his professional career as an engineer. His respect for scientific data, and his skill in analyzing data, are based on that background. Dr. Colgan also has extensive training in psychology and physiology. His research on the relationship of nutrition to health and behavior has benefited greatly by this nontraditional background. The findings he reports are based on a computer analysis (he built his own computer!) of hundreds of cases from his clinics at the University of Auckland in New Zealand and at The Rockefeller University in New York City.

Michael Colgan is by no means the first to emphasize the strong link between nutrition and vitality. Many excellent physicians and scientists have studied the matter and have reported their findings in lectures, books and articles. What has attracted international recognition of Dr. Colgan's work is the remarkable improvements in performance he has brought about in highly trained athletes, such as marathon runners and weight lifters. Now we have hard data, from carefully controlled studies. The runners, already in peak condition, one would think, have trimmed an average of seventeen minutes off their best times while on high levels of nutrients. Similarly, the weight lifters set new personal records while on the high-level nutrients, only to have their performances decline again during the placebo phase of the studies.

Others have worked with athletes, but usually their experiments have involved one or two nutrients at a time, and only in moderate amounts. Colgan has boldly broken with this tradition in his attempt to see what nutrients in *optimum* quantities can achieve. Colgan's emphasis on the importance of using the *full range* of available nutrients also sets him apart. He stresses *synergy,* the working together of the vitamins and minerals in an integrated way. And he produces *results,* not only in athletes, but in all people who seek higher levels of vitality, effectiveness and longevity.

Colgan is not content merely to research and preach; he actually practices what he preaches. He is an accomplished marathon runner, and is able to perform one-arm chin-ups and push-ups. An unusual academic indeed.

Dr. Colgan's work will be acclaimed by the many open-minded, nutritionally oriented physicians and scientists who applaud important new developments, irrespective of the damage these new developments may do to established traditions and beliefs. Dr. Colgan's work will be roundly criticized by many other people, particularly by the typical establishment physician (TEP), who has a strong vested interest in the status quo, and who will not examine evidence contrary to his training and beliefs. Despite the mountains of scientific references and other forms of scientific data provided by Dr. Colgan, the TEP will continue to assert that "there is no scientific evidence to support that view." I have encountered many such physicians, and when they say, "There is no scientific evidence," they mean merely, "I haven't taken trouble to look for any scientific evidence, and I find it much more convenient to continue to insist that there is no such evidence than to bother to look at it."

The TEP is trained in the use of drugs. He is, after all, as the gold lettering on his door indicates, a doctor of *medicine.* His specialty is medicine—drugs—and not nutrition. It should therefore not be surprising that he would know little or nothing about nutrition, for the most part, and would be rather hostile to the idea that nutrition can bring about better health and functioning than can be brought about by the drugs he prescribes. After all, if you are not up on something, you are likely to be down on it.

Ironically, the public looks to the medical establishment for information and advice on nutrition. I have given numerous talks at medical schools, and these typically are scheduled for the lunch hour. I am appalled at the number of white-coated physicians and physicians-in-training in these audiences whose "lunch" consists of a soft drink and a sack of potato chips.

Nevertheless, despite the strong, and expected, opposition from the medical establishment, a new era is dawning. The public is becoming very much aware of the dangers of the drug-oriented approach to health. They are becoming aware of the fact that Mother Nature is far more clever than we, and that we must learn about the functioning of the body—and the natural substances, such as vitamins and minerals, that the body uses—if we are to have any hope of assisting nature in bringing about optimum functioning. Dr. Colgan's work, as presented in this book, goes a long way toward bringing us to that understanding, and making it possible for us to use the latest findings of scientific and nutritional research in our quest for health, longevity and optimum performance.

—BERNARD RIMLAND, PH.D.

San Diego, California
June 22, 1982

ACKNOWLEDGMENTS

So MANY people have formulated my thoughts. So many are with me in the task of preventing degenerative disease. I can name only a fraction of them. Stuart Slater, mentor extraordinaire, taught me what I am, though I still cannot fully comprehend it. Dr. John Irwin, my boss at the University of Auckland, maintained a sneaking faith in me when others doubted. Dr. Linus Pauling's prompt and gracious correspondence gave me the necessary confidence. Through his writings I have been privileged to glimpse that rare compassion for humanity which has set me on my present road. Dr. Bernard Rimland's pioneering work in nutritional treatment of autistic children first convinced me in 1972 that the "good mixed diet" is anything but, and can cause serious illness. Similarly, Dr. Carl Pfeiffer, physician and scholar, showed me how a deficiency of even one essential mineral makes optimum health impossible. Through his books and papers swiftly and courteously sent, Dr. Roger Williams taught me the principles of biochemical individuality. Dr. Michael Brines, my colleague at Rockefeller University, gentle scholar, always seems to know everything before I do. Dr. Neal Miller, my boss at Rockefeller, tolerated my radical views and gave me more time to write them. Dr. Jonas Salk, whose courage and brilliance have saved countless millions from polio, with one sentence showed me how to change the direction of this book (and all my other work) so that it might better benefit the health of Americans. With bubbling enthusiasm and meticulous editing, Elizabeth Frost Knappman, my editor at Morrow, pushed me through the four hectic months of writing. Finally, special gratitude goes to my wife, my love, Lesley, who has blossomed over eight wonderful years into my best mentor, friend, companion. Somebody up there must like me to have assigned such a lovely guardian angel.

Despite their help, or perhaps because of it, I am solely responsible for all conclusions herein.

CONTENTS

ONE: VITAMINS AND MINERALS FOR OPTIMUM HEALTH

TWO: FOUR BIG KILLERS AND LOTS OF LITTLE ONES

SECTION ONE

Vitamins and Minerals for Optimum Health

CHAPTER 1

HOW HEALTHY ARE WE?

THE SURGEON GENERAL tells us Americans have never been healthier. True, medical science has beaten most infectious diseases and can lessen the symptoms of many others. But these advances have left us prey to worse fates, degenerative diseases such as cardiovascular disease, cancer and diabetes. Dr. Robert Levy, director of the National Heart, Lung and Blood Institute, reports that 35 million Americans suffer from hypertension, a major cause of the 500,000 strokes and 1.25 million heart attacks each year.[1] Cancer prospects are even worse. Despite television theatricals praising the effectiveness of cancer treatments, the National Cancer Institute reported in 1981 that one in every three Americans will get cancer before the age of seventy-four.[2] That's one third of our population! Does this sound like better health than our forefathers?

From 1960 to 1978 the cost of American medical care mushroomed from $27 billion to $192 billion a year.[3] Despite this incredible offering, the degenerative diseases remain hungrier than ever. In order of importance in causing death and disability they are:

Heart disease
Other cardiovascular diseases
Hypertension
Cancers

Mental disorders (including alcoholism and drug misuse)
Diabetes
Arthritis
Obesity
Hypoglycemia
Hypothyroidism

Together these afflictions cause eight of every ten deaths in America.[4] The amount of suffering they produce is incalculable. Though they appear quite different from each other, all have the same basis, the progressive degeneration of bodily systems because of cumulative effects of illnesses, injuries, bodily pollution and malnutrition over many years. But through the system described in this book most are preventable.

Medical Treatment Is NOT the Answer

The main reason medicine is failing with the degenerative diseases is its concentration on treatment after illness has struck. Most of our health money is directed to *treatment* rather than prevention. Only four cents in each health dollar are spent on preventive medicine.[5] This bias toward treatment offers too little, too late. The degenerative diseases listed are all manifestations of general systemic disorders which develop years before the symptoms get bad enough to notice or to bring you to a physician. Many times symptoms do not appear at all until the disease is in a terminal stage. In heart disease the first symptom is often an attack that kills. Such attacks do not happen to healthy hearts. As with cancer, most heart disease may grow insidiously for a decade with no symptoms at all. It is not surprising that medicine fails if the first opportunity to treat comes when half or more of a vital organ system is already dead or replaced by malignant growths.

Nevertheless, treatment is still the popular approach. A lifesaving operation seems more real and deserving of medical (and media) attention than the nonoccurrence of a disease. Yet the history of medicine in Western society shows that the treatment of illness has *never* been the key to reducing its incidence. Professor René Dubos of Rockefeller University, for example, shows that the rate of tuberculosis in New York City had fallen by 75 percent *before* the first sanatorium was opened in 1910. Treatment of the disease had nothing to do with this improvement. The disappearance of most tuberculosis was a direct result of improvements in nutrition, living conditions and sanitation. These, especially improved nutrition, increased the resistance of individuals to the disease and prevented them from developing it.[6]

Similarly, the eradication of diarrhea had little to do with its medical treatment. Formerly a major cause of infant death in America and Britain, diarrhea killed 170 babies in every 1,000 in New York City in the 1890's. Then, over the next ten years a succession of health-conscious mayors made major improvements in street sanitation, milk sterilization, garbage disposal and the establishment of parks and recreation areas. By 1902 infant deaths from diarrhea had been cut by half to eighty-five per thousand.[7] Clean milk, clean streets and fresh air saved those children by making them generally healthier and more resistant to disease.

The same is true for diphtheria, whooping cough, scarlet fever, mumps and measles. With improvements in living conditions, sanitation and nutrition, the combined death rate from all these diseases had dwindled to one fifth of what it was in the early part of this century, long *before* the advent of immunization and antibiotics.[8] Polio is another example. Like measles, it finally succumbed to advances in medical science after the introduction of vaccines for both diseases in the late 1950's and early 1960's. But these diseases were not conquered by *treatment* of patients who had them, but rather by immunization to prevent them from happening. Like good nutrition, immunization is a preventive strategy which increases host resistance. The

Surgeon General agrees: "Nearly all the gains against the once-great killers have come as a result of improvements in sanitation, housing, nutrition and immunization."[9]

Medicine Does NOT Promote Prevention

Most American hospitals are built for treatment, *not* for prevention. They have neither the equipment nor the procedures to prevent disease, and most physicians have no training in this area. Until there is a radical reorganization of hospitals and of medical education, medicine cannot use health money effectively. The hospital treatment armamentarium built from Pasteur's discoveries that microbes cause infections is powerless against the noninfective degenerative diseases. Immunization cannot help either, because these diseases have no infective agents against which vaccines could protect us. This leaves housing, sanitation and nutrition as weapons against disease. Clearly, combating degenerative disease is no longer the physicians' battle. It is ours. As the Surgeon General says, "You, the individual, can do more for your own health and well-being than any doctor, any hospital, any drug, any exotic medical device."[10]

The first step in assuming responsibility for your well-being is to learn the facts and the risks concerning health. This is hard, since many sources of health information do not promote health but serve the vested interests that finance them. It does not promote medicine, for example, to tell the public of the huge, well-documented and disgraceful state of hospital malnutrition in America, caused directly by hospital diets."[11] And it does not help a hospital equipment company's sales to let you know that their astronomically expensive coronary care units do not extend the lives of heart-attack patients.[12] Nor do television promotions of the pharmaceutical industry mention the harmful side effects of their drugs.[13] You must learn to protect yourself against the maze of health misinformation.

Life Expectancy Is NOT Improving

How long we live is often used as a measure of the effectiveness of medicine. Doctors are proud that the average life expectancy of a baby born in American today is seventy-three years (and a bit), whereas in 1900 it was only forty-seven years. So now we enjoy an additional twenty-six years of life. What is seldom revealed, however, is that almost all this increase took place before 1949. By then, average life expectancy had already risen by twenty-one years, to sixty-eight years (and a bit).[14] And this huge improvement occurred without the benefit of mass immunization, antibiotics or the supertechnology of modern hospitals.

Most of the increase in life expectancy came from reducing infant mortality, not from reducing disease in adults. Every baby who dies at birth drastically reduces average life expectancy. For example, if we take one hundred people who live to age eighty, then their average life is eighty years. If we take one hundred babies who die at birth (age zero), then their average life is zero years. Taking the two hundred together, the total years lived for the combined group is: 100 (babies) × 0 (years old) + 100 (adults) × 80 (years old) = 8,000 years. To get the average length of life, we divide the total years lived by the number of persons. That is 8,000/200, which equals *40 years.* The babies who died at birth have halved the life expectancy figure. So, calculating life expectancy from birth on can be deceiving.

In 1900 many babies died in infancy, so the average life expectancy looked very low. Once past childhood, however, people lived nearly as long as they do now. If we ask what our life expectancy as adults is in comparison to our forebears, most of the apparent gains disappear. In 1920 a twenty-five-year-old white male American had a remaining life expectancy of forty-six years, almost the same as a twenty-five-year-old today. His father, at age fifty in 1920, had a remaining life expectancy of twenty-two years, almost the same as a fifty-year-old today. For an adult aged sixty-five, life expectancy has increased by only four years since 1900, and nearly all of that is an extension in the life of women.[15] So, the twenty-six-year extension of life calculated from figures for infants is illusory for every one of us. Despite kidney cleaners, pacemakers, heart transplants and life-support machines, on the average, you and I still stubbornly die at seventy-three.

Clearly, the mountain of money being gulped by medical technology is ill spent. In the 1920's medical costs were a minute fraction of the American economy.[16] Now, "the disease industry" is the second largest industry in the United States.[17] Yet the health of Americans, measured by length of life, is not improving. Between 1960 and 1980, when more money was poured into medical treatment than ever before, life expectancy did not increase at all. In fact, as infant deaths declined, deaths of adults *increased.* The net result is a three months' *decline* in life expectancy since 1960. In April 1981 an American male infant had a worse life expectancy than the infants of twenty-three other countries, including countries with harsh climates, such as Iceland, or poor medical care, such as Greece, Spain and Puerto Rico.[18] Perhaps other measures of health will be more encouraging.

Health Expectancy Is NOT Improving Either

Of course, length of life is not synonymous with quality of life. As one measure of quality we can look for improvements in the quality of our health care. Hospitals, the center of American medicine, take the largest and the fastest-growing bite from our health dollars. In the early 1960's hospital charges rose at about 7 percent a year. Then, in 1965, anticipating the income from Medicaid and Medicare beginning in 1966, charges suddenly ballooned to double in the next five years. So, this area should be showing big improvements. Unfortunately, there is no evidence whatsoever that the health of patients has been improved.[19]

On the contrary, the large hospital complexes common in the United States, Britain and Europe are only marginally useful in health care. Bureaucratic complexities, personnel shortages, escalating costs, ignorance of preventive measures and restricted access to effective treatment are canceling the gains of medical science.[20] Worse, organizational developments are transforming many patients into pawns of the disease industry. David Kotelchuck, editor of the Health Policy Advisory Center book *Prognosis Negative,* shows how many hospitals have become commercial enterprises complete with stockholders, growth targets and profit motives. No matter how skilled and dedicated, their physicians are increasingly subjected to the dictates of corporate goals. Profitable bed-occupancy rates as a criterion of hospital success are hardly compatible with medicine's aim to discharge the patient in good health as quickly as possible.

This sad decline of ethics has been well documented.[21] For instance, seven out of every ten malpractice suits are for problems in hospitals. After thorough investigation, in 1973 the United States Department of Health, Education and Welfare concluded that it is not merely physicians who are at fault, but defects in hospital administration, defects in hospital technology and inherent dangers of modern hospital environments.[22] Today one in every five patients admitted to American hospitals is likely to suffer additional illness or injury as a direct result of his or her hospitalization.[23]

These risks are not confined to America. Exactly the same 20 percent risk of iatrogenic illness (illness caused by hospital, physician or treatment) was found in 1977 by the New South Wales Health Commission survey of its hospitals in Australia. This survey also examined the efficacy of hospital treatment by checking with discharged patients. Nearly half the patients reported that their condition had not been improved at all by the hospital treatment, and 10 percent were worse after hospitalization than before it.[24] So, if we take these hospitals as average, hospital treatment offers a less than 50 percent chance of curing illness, and a significant chance of leaving you sicker.

This is not too surprising when you consider that most hospitalization is now for the chronic degenerative diseases, against which medical treatment is ineffective. Cardiovascular disease, cancer and mental degeneration now claim more hospital beds than all other illnesses combined. Despite their fine and dedicated service to many individuals, the vastly expensive development of hospitals in recent years is inappropriate and ineffective against the new pestilence.

There are other signs of slippage in the state of Western health. Not counting patients in hospitals and institutions, one person in every eight in America now has a chronic disabling condition limiting his or her life and activity.[25] Eight people in every ten over the age of sixty-five have at least one chronic condition.[26] And the major degenerative diseases are more than holding their own against medicine. Even with bypass surgery, electronic gee-whiz and daily pharmaceutical "miracles," you are just as likely to die of a heart attack as in 1910.[27] You are nine times more likely to have heart disease than a Japanese,[28] and no one would charge that American medicine is only one ninth as effective as Japanese medicine. Our environment and nutrition are the culprits, because Japanese who move to the United States quickly change to develop heart disease as frequently as Americans.[29] Despite our spending more on health per capita than any country on earth, twenty-six other countries now have a lower death rate from cardiovascular disease.[30]

As the Surgeon General says, cancer death rates are increasing, most cancers are caused by environmental and nutritional pollution, and prevention is our major solution.[31] Twenty-five other countries now do better than America in preventing cancer.[32] Diabetes is also increasing, and insulin treatment is now known to be an answer only to diabetic coma. Unless controlled by nutrition, the disease progresses inexorably, often to gangrene, blindness and cardiovascular disease.[33]

As a final example, the President's Commission on Mental Health estimates that a quarter of the American population, that is, *one in every four people passing you on the street,* is now suffering from depression, anxiety or other emotional disorders.[34] The suicide rate among young people (fifteen to twenty-four years old) is *five times* what it was in 1950.[35] Now, one in every ten deaths in this age group is a suicide, strong evidence of the declining mental health of American youth. Even in the very young, the future of American society, mental problems are increasing. Even allowing for the improvement in detection and classification, since 1960 there has still been a huge rise in the number of children with brain damage, hyperactivity or learning disability of unknown origin. Now, almost one child in every five is affected.[36] A study now in progress at the University of California suggests that the problem has doubled since the 1960's.[37]

America is not alone in this declining health trend. Similar declines have occurred in Britain and France, both of which have made a massive effort to improve medical treatment over the past twenty years. Even the rich, comfortable welfare state of Sweden recognizes that its overall health has not improved since the 1950's. The National Swedish Board of Health and Welfare reports that today every third Swedish child has mental problems. Every third Swedish adult, male and female, suffers from sleep disorders, depression or anxiety.[38]

The reliance on medical treatment to reduce disease is dependence on an ineffectual resource. As we shall see, the tragedy is that much disease is preventable. And the means of prevention do not involve medical supertechnology, but are simple, straightforward and within the understanding and the wallet of all of us.

CHAPTER 2

THE MYTH OF THE GOOD MIXED DIET

MANY CLAIM THAT America has nutritious foods in abundance and that everyone gets adequate nutrition by eating a good mixed diet. This may have been true at one time, when people grew much of their own food or bought it from local growers. But with modern methods of storage and processing, our food comes from all over the world and may be *years* old before we get to eat it. As we will see, this food can be completely devoid of nutrients and may also contain harmful chemicals that have no business in the human body.

Even if the foods *were* adequate, most people don't know what constitutes a good mixed diet, and even fewer actually eat it. Dr. Victor Herbert is typical of the nutrition scientists who believe that the good mixed diet provides adequate nutrition and that it is easy to obtain. He recommends that *each day* you eat "a wide variety of foods from each of the four food groups (grains, fruits and vegetables, meats, and milk)." More specifically, he states that *each day* you should eat four portions of fruits and vegetables (including one uncooked), two portions of meat, fish, poultry or eggs, and two or three portions of milk and milk products.[1]

That's a lot of food. But apart from making the nation even fatter than it is already, it is pie-in-the-sky advice. First, Dr. Herbert makes no allowance for the absence of nutrients in much of our food today. Second, social and occupational pressures of modern life make it impossible for most of us to follow such a regimen. Contrast his advice with the cereal-and-toast breakfast, the fast-food lunch and the restaurant dinner that are an obligatory way of life for many urban dwellers. If my analysis is correct, that we get neither the nutrients nor the good mixed diet, there should be abundant evidence of nutritional deficiency in America. Let's see.

Americans ARE Malnourished

Authorities began to suspect the nutritional state of America in the 1960's. But it was 1971 before anything substantial was done to measure it. The first Health and Nutrition Examination Survey (HANES 1) ran from May 1971 to June 1974 under congressional mandate by the National Health Survey Act. It studied twenty-eight thousand people, from age one to age seventy-four, in sixty-five different areas throughout the United States.[2] HANES 1 examined the diets people actually ate, the levels of nutrients in their blood and any symptoms of malnutrition. Using very conservative levels as the norm, it found huge dietary deficiencies. For instance, nine women out of every ten had insufficient iron in their diets (less than 18 mg). One in every two women had insufficient calcium (less than 600 mg). Iron deficiency in the blood was widespread in all age, sex, race and income groups, despite the fact that white bread and cereals in America are "enriched" with iron. As we will see, simply putting one or another nutrient back into foods is useless. It is the interactions of multiple nutrients that determine their capacity for absorption and utilization by the body. Overall, more than 60 percent of these people showed at least one symptom of malnutrition, regardless of their income level.

This study confirmed the findings of the larger Ten State Nutritional Survey of eighty-six thousand people who were mainly on lower incomes.[3] To take a few examples from this survey, in Michigan more than half the men and women tested were deficient in folic acid. In Texas and Washington one in every four men and one in every three women were deficient in Vitamin A. One in three persons in southern California was deficient in Vitamin B_2 (riboflavin). In Texas 10 percent of persons were deficient in Vitamin C and 10 percent were deficient in Vitamin B_1. And these figures took very low values as representing adequate nutrition. If the norms used in this book were taken, almost everyone would have been judged deficient. Nevertheless, even using conservative norms, about two thirds of these people were malnourished even though the number of nutrients tested for deficiency was only a quarter of the forty-nine nutrients essential for health.

These problems are not confined to the United States. In Canada, for example, a survey of twenty-one thousand people (including the Eskimo and Indian samples) showed that seven out of every ten men and six out of every ten women were deficient in folic acid, a quarter of the men and women were deficient in Vitamin C, a third of the women were iron deficient, and a third of the men and a fifth of the women were thiamine deficient. Eskimos and Indians showed worse deficiencies.[4] And remember, these figures are based on a norm consisting of the *minimum* amounts of vitamins required to prevent disease, not the amounts necessary for good health. Deficiencies need not be at the level of producing obvious disease in order to be injurious.

If you are still not convinced that nutritional deficiencies are widespread, then let's examine one place that should be able to provide a diet that is nutritionally adequate: the hospital. Unfortunately, we find just the opposite. Recent studies have revealed widespread malnutrition in these expensive institutions. It started in 1965, when Dr. C. M. Leevy found vitamin deficiencies in a ramdom sample of patients in a major municipal hospital.[5] There followed similar findings of poor nutritional status in patients in another hospital reported in the *American Journal of Clinical Nutrition* by Drs. A. J. Bollet and S. Owens.[6] By 1974 there was a flood of reports. Dr. Bruce Bistrian found moderate to severe protein and calorie malnutrition in *half* the surgical patients of a Boston municipal hospital.[7] Respected authority on nutrition Dr. C. E. Butterworth discovered that thirty of fifty-six patients became malnourished *after* their admission to the hospital, and *not* as a direct result of their illness.[8]

Very likely these people were deprived of good nutrition because of the poor nutritional content of the hospital food.[9] Dr. Butterworth wrote in his editorial column in the *Journal of the American Medical Association* in 1974:

> The time has come to reevaluate current practices and standards with regard to the nutritional care of hospitalized patients. It makes no sense to spend vast sums in technologically complex areas while neglecting such a fundamentally important subject as nutrition. . . . The conclusion seems inescapable that the systems necessary to provide comprehensive nutritional care for hospitalized patients are lagging far behind other areas. A major burden of responsibility must fall on the shoulders of the physician. His deficiencies in turn are the inevitable consequence of the longstanding neglect of nutrition education in our medical schools.[10]

Dr. Butterworth's plea fell on deaf ears. Since 1974 even more disturbing evidence has surfaced. In 1979 Dr. Leslie Klevay, a world authority on mineral requirements in nutrition, found serious mineral deficiencies in hospital diets of the Medical Center Rehabilitation Hospital in North Dakota.[11] Further studies by Dr. Bruce Bistrian and his colleagues found serious malnutrition in both medical and surgical patients at Boston City Hospital. They concluded it was not only that particular hospital which is at fault but that such malnutrition occurs commonly in municipal hospitals.[12] Dr. Maurice Shils, director of clinical nutrition at the Sloan-Kettering Cancer Hospital in New York, told the World Nutrition Congress in 1980 that often by the time a nutrition consultant is called in, patients have already become seriously malnourished.[13]

As a final example, Dr. Roland Weinsier and his colleagues

at the University of Alabama measured the nutritional status of 134 patients on admission to a major Alabama hospital. During their treatment more than 75 percent of the patients became malnourished. The longer their stay, the worse their nutritional status became, increasing their risk of death and prolonging their hospitalization.[14] These investigators concluded that many hospitals would show a similar pattern. So, if anything, hospital malnutrition has been getting worse. If our hospitals can't provide adequate diets with all their resources, dieticians, nutritionists and specialists, it is very unlikely you can get one by selection from the supermarket shelf.

The latest findings on malnutrition in the general population show that the worsening trend in hospitals is also occurring in homes across the nation. The Nationwide Food Consumption Survey of 1977–1978, by the U.S. Department of Agriculture (USDA), measured nutrients in foods used in a week in fifteen thousand households.[15] One in every three households had diets deficient in calcium and Vitamin B_6. One in every four was deficient in magnesium. One in five was deficient in iron and Vitamin A. The diets of teenage girls were seriously deficient in calcium, iron, magnesium and Vitamin B_6. And the standards taken as normal were the very conservative Recommended Daily Allowances (RDAs). No extra allowances were made for the destruction of nutrients by food processing and cooking. No allowances were made either for the increased nutrients required in pregnancy, lactation, illness or stress. For the pregnant among these girls, their babies risk birth deformity, mental retardation, congenital diseases or low birth weight with all its attendant hazards. It is sad to see such evidence when these problems are so easily preventable. Against all this evidence from the nutrition surveys, the hospitals and the food survey, *if anyone tells you that Americans get adequate nourishment from their "good mixed diet"—don't believe them.*

You Don't Know Whether Your Food Is Nutritious

You can't even find out what is in your food. Since 1973, in my own clinic in Auckland, New Zealand, in another clinic at Auckland University and in a local hospital, we began to take note of symptoms of malnourishment. Soon we were finding that three quarters of the patients had at least one sign of malnutrition. Some had many signs. None showed outright deficiency diseases, but there were clear symptoms, both clinical and biochemical. Yet when we listed their daily food, almost all the patients seemed to be on the mythical good mixed diet. Then we began to measure the vitamin and mineral contents of some of the foods they actually ate. We were amazed to find that even fresh, raw foods did not contain anything like the amounts of nutrients given in nutrition tables.

Just as you do when buying your food, we bought a wide variety of common foods from numerous different suppliers. On testing raw carrots, for example, we found that different samples of 100 g (3½ oz) varied in Provitamin A content from 70 IU to 18,500 IU. So, if we take the Recommended Daily Allowance (RDA) of 5,000 IU as a minimum standard, then eating carrots every day could result in either a completely inadequate supply of Vitamin A or an overabundance, *depending on the carrots.*

Wheat germ varied also. Fresh samples of 100 g varied in Vitamin E content from 3.2 IU to 21 IU. So you cannot rely on wheat germ to provide your Vitamin E. Different brands of stone-ground whole wheat flour varied so widely in content of Vitamin B complex that it was meaningless to calculate an average value. Pantothenic acid, for example, ranged between 0.3 mg and 3.3 mg per 100 g, an elevenfold variation. The ranges for other common foods tested are shown in Tables 1 to 4. The American Medical Association and the U.S. Department of Agriculture have published similar findings.[16]

Today, when we know nothing about what has happened to

Table 1: Variations in Vitamin A Content of Common Foods Reputedly High in Vitamin A Value (per 100 g of fresh raw food)

	Calf Liver	*Carrots (unpeeled)*	*Tomatoes (with skin)*	*White Cheddar Cheese*	*Eggs (without shell)*
Vitamin A and Provitamin A Content (IU)	470–41,200	70–18,500	640–3,020	735–1,590	905–1,220

Table 2: Variations in Vitamin C Content of Common Foods Reputedly High in Vitamin C Value (per 100 g of fresh raw food)

	Oranges (without skin)	*Tomatoes (with skin)*	*Calf Liver*	*Carrots (unpeeled)*
Vitamin C (mg)	Trace–116	9–38	15–36	1–8

Table 3: Variations in Vitamin E Content of Common Foods Reputedly High in Vitamin E Value (per 100 g of fresh raw food)

	Wheat Germ	*Stone-ground Whole Wheat Flour*	*Carrots (unpeeled)*
Vitamin E (IU)	3.2–21.0	0.8–9.8	Trace–1.6

Table 4: Variations in B Complex Vitamins in Common Foods Reputedly High in B Complex Value (per 100 g of fresh raw food)

	Wheat Germ	*Calf Liver*	*Stone-ground Whole Wheat Flour*
B_1 Thiamine (mg)	0.7–2.1	Trace–0.4	Trace–0.6
B_2 Riboflavin (mg)	0.5–1.7	1.0–3.6	(No tests done)
B_3 Niacin (mg)	2.0–5.5	8.5–13.4	2.9–7.0
B_5 Pantothenic acid (mg)	0.9–4.0	5.2–8.8	0.3–3.3
B_6 Pyridoxine (mg)	0.8–1.1	0.5–0.7	Trace–0.4
B_{12} Cobalamin (mcg)	(No tests done)	55–82	(No tests done)
Folic acid (mcg)	109–362	201–313	33–149

the food we eat after it is harvested or killed, there is no way we can know its nutrient content. The first oranges we tested were bought from a local supermarket. Their Vitamin C content was zero. They looked, smelled and tasted perfectly normal. Probably they had been stored for a long time. Similar oranges we bought directly from the grower, picked that day, contained 180 mg of Vitamin C per orange (116 mg/100 g)—a very healthy amount. Nutrition tables often give 80 mg as the Vitamin C content of an average orange. We found the range to vary between zero and 180 mg. This gives an *average* Vitamin C content of 90 mg per orange, not too different from the table. But the average is meaningless if you want to know how much Vitamin C you are getting from your freshly squeezed orange juice. Depending on the orange, you could be getting a lot—or none at all! Such enormous variations in the nutrient content of even raw foods make nonsense of advice that a good mixed diet provides ample nutrition. They also make nonsense of tables of nutrients in food given in many diet and nutrition books.

The essential mineral content of foods varies even more widely than the vitamin content. The mineral selenium, for example, essential for proper functioning of the heart, is deficient in the soils in many parts of the world. The selenium in crops and in livestock raised on the soils varies likewise. In the United States the selenium content of some crops varies by a factor of 200.[17] Even the wheat that makes your bread can contain anything from 50 mcg to 800 mcg of selenium per kilo (2¼ lbs). We take 200 mcg as the minimum adult norm. A daily diet containing half a pound or so of whole wheat bread (6–8 slices) contains anything from an adequate 200 mcg of selenium down to a dangerously deficient 12.5 mcg.

Variations in mineral content of soils and crops are so vital to health that no farmer today would consider trying to raise top-grade livestock without supplementing their feed. You don't get champion racehorses either without careful supplementation. Yet the government vacillates to the beck and call of the food lobbies, leaving us humans to fend for ourselves, despite the undeniable evidence that the mineral content of our food is an important determinant of resistance to disease.[18] The enormous variations in mineral content of water and soils and the foods that grow in and on them make tables of average mineral contents of foods useless for calculating your own intake. *Unless you take a mineral supplement, there is no way you can know how much or how little you are getting.*

It is not only the variations in foods that confound us, but also what has been done to the foods. Those we test are fresh, unprocessed and raw. Meat is bought from the slaughterhouse, slaughtered that day. Apart from the supermarket oranges, fruit and vegetables are bought directly from the growers. Flour and wheat germ are bought from the mills. Most of us do not get food that fresh. Our daily bread is stale by comparison, so it is likely to be much less nutritious. For example, lettuce stored at room temperature loses 50 percent of its Vitamin C in twenty-four hours after picking. Keeping it in the refrigerator results in the same loss in three days.[19] More stable vegetables, such as asparagus, broccoli and green beans, also lose 50 percent of their Vitamin C in cold storage before they reach your greengrocer.[20] Cooking vegetables destroys another 25 percent of the Vitamin C and up to 70 percent of the thiamine and 50 percent of the riboflavin. And these are what we call "fresh" vegetables.

If foods are processed in any way, they lose far more nutrients before reaching your table. Dr. Henry Schroeder, the foremost American authority on nutrient content of food, analyzed 730 common foods.[21] To take just a few examples, canning of green vegetables destroys more than 50 percent of Vitamin B_5 and B_6. Canning of peas and beans destroys more than 75 percent of the same vitamins. Essential minerals are not saved either. Canning of carrots removes 70 percent of the cobalt, canning of tomatoes removes 80 percent of the zinc. The lists are endless. And if the cans are stored for a long time, about another 25 percent of the vitamin content is lost.[22] Freezing is a little better but still destroys over half the B vitamins. Freezing of meat, for example, destroys 70 percent of the B_5. Remember, these are not rough estimates, but careful measures over many tests. And none of these lost vitamins are added back into the foods after processing. So, if you use canned or frozen foods or eat in restaurants, almost all of which use them extensively, you are getting only the meager leftovers of nutrients.

It is easy to see why hospital diets are deficient when they are planned from tables of average nutrient contents of foods. Unless hospital dieticians measure the content of each item, which is completely impractical, they can no more know what is in the food than you or I. After much testing in our clinics, we came to the reluctant conclusion that the only sure way to know what patients were getting was to give them vitamin and mineral supplements whose nutrient content is known and unchanging. Remember, these supplements are not drugs. Drugs are substances foreign to the body, which it attempts to eliminate as quickly as possible. Vitamins and essential minerals are nutrients, integral components of the body structure developed over millions of years of evolution to keep it in optimal condition. Without them you will die.

Food Pollution and the Principle of Synergy

Everyone in nutrition science knows the health value of eating fresh whole foods and avoiding processed junk. We constantly barrage the public with such advice. But how many of us follow it? It is a source of constant bewilderment for me at conferences to sit at a table of distinguished nutrition scientists and watch them eat rubbish bread, chemically treated meat, overstewed vegetables and sugar and starch desserts, just because that is all that's offered, and it's free with the conference package. Every time I attend such conferences, I hope for a person of sufficient conviction to leap up and denounce us. It never happens. At one of the most famous universities in the world for nutrition research (whose name I had better not mention), I "brown bag" it for lunch because there is no decent food in the restaurant. My colleagues comment, "Beyond our control," "It's an outside concession," or "It's worse at the hospital!"

We have become a nation of convenience eaters. Since 1960 we have increased our consumption of soft drinks per person by 160 percent. Each year, we now drink five hundred glasses of these beverages apiece. We have increased our use of frozen vegetables over fresh vegetables by 400 percent, and our use of corn syrup by over 200 percent in the same period. Use of fresh fruits and vegetables has declined steadily since 1920. We now eat 70 percent fewer apples per person, 74 percent fewer fresh potatoes, 65 percent less fresh cabbage.[23] Today two thirds of the average diet is highly processed "food."[24]

Most patients in our clinics and participants in our experiments ate a large proportion of processed foods in their diets. Some of these contained very few nutrients at all. White bread, for example, loses most of its nutrients in the processing of grain into white flour. This ubiquitous "food" is so devoid of the elements essential for life that even weevils cannot live on it. So-called enriched white flour is little better. Although it has thiamine, riboflavin, niacin, plus calcium and iron, added back, it has lost its pantothenic acid, pyridoxine, folic acid, Vitamin E, magnesium, zinc, copper and manganese.

To explain why these losses are important it is necessary to introduce the first principle of my system for determining nutritional needs—*the rule of synergy.* Because of the way your body has evolved, no single nutrient can do anything for your health. *It is the multiple interactions of nutrients,* NOT their single actions, which are the basis of their biological functions. This principle has been only recently emphasized in nutrition science,[25] although top scientists have known it for many years. Until the advent of powerful laboratory computers in the last decade, it wasn't possible to do the complex analyses that have made the truth obvious. Unfortunately, much medical advice on nutrition and even the Recommended Daily Allowances (RDAs) are based largely on obsolete, single-nutrient experiments, often done *in vitro* (in the test tube) outside the body. These studies have little relevance to the function of nutrients in the human system. Single actions of nutrients are secondary and often unimportant. It is the multiple interactions, the *synergy* of nutrients that count.

Let us apply this principle to "enriched" bread. The human body evolved over millions of years, ingesting seeds, grains and plants containing certain complexes of nutrients. By the natural selection process of evolution, the body developed the mechanisms necessary to use these nutrients simultaneously, each one being essential in a chain of interactions. Only in this century has technology enabled us to make grain and cereal products that have been stripped of their nutrients. Such products have never occurred in nature, and therefore the body has never had the opportunity to develop mechanisms to deal with them. We have the same digestive system, the same biochemical system, as our ancestors. Evolution is very slow. Perhaps in another hundred thousand years we could develop mechanisms that would enable us to survive on white flour carbohydrate. Today we cannot.

For example, even the basic textbooks of biochemistry tell us that the simple metabolism of carbohydrate, disregarding all its other functions, requires niacin, thiamine, riboflavin, pantothenic acid, pyridoxine, phosphorus and magnesium.[26] The last four of these nutrients are lost in milling white flour *and are not added back.* Yet if any one of them is missing, the carbohydrate cannot be used by the body. In order to use "enriched" bread, the body must rob itself, depriving heart and bone of phosphorus and magnesium, depriving nerve and muscle of pantothenic acid, depriving blood and brain of pyridoxine. And still we wonder about our epidemic of degenerative disease!

The inability of the mammal system to deal with "enriched" bread is demonstrated in some important experiments by Professor Roger Williams and his colleagues at the University of Texas. Sixty-four rats were fed "enriched" bread from weaning on. After three months two thirds of them had died and the rest had growth abnormalities.[27] A control group, fed the same bread but with the addition of vitamins, minerals and amino acids to make it nutritious, thrived. In another study rats fed on ordinary commercial white bread died in sixty days.[28] If this "food" cannot support the life of a rat, a very tough, adaptable creature, then it certainly cannot support the life of a human child. If you feed your baby a lot of white bread, it is certain you are inhibiting the child's development and laying the foundation for degenerative disease later in life. Use whole grain bread instead and start a healthy food habit that will continue to help the child throughout life.

We Still Eat Too Much Salt

Processing adds huge amounts of unnecessary salt to our food. Americans now eat twenty times the salt needed for good health.[29] You can read about salt's causative links with hypertension in Chapter 9. It is the sodium in salt that does the damage. Canned carrots, for example, have five times the sodium of raw carrots. Canned peas have *one hundred times* the sodium of raw peas. Next time your adrenalin has you gobbling popcorn at a movie thriller, remember that the average commercial salted popcorn contains *six hundred times* the sodium of plain popcorn.[30]

Thanks to the nutrition lobby, the practice of adding salt to baby foods is disappearing. Mother's milk contains 16 mg sodium per 100 g. Canned baby foods can contain *300 mg per 100 g,* twelve times as much. If infants needed all that salt, nature would have provided it at the breast. Even if we consider the ingredients in canned baby foods, the canning process can add five times the sodium that occurs naturally in the meats and up to two hundred times the sodium that occurs naturally in the cereal and vegetables.[31] At present it is still not proven that salt-loading predisposes a child to hypertension, though it certainly produces hypertension in adults.[32] With over thirty million of the hypertensives in America having no known physical cause for their disease except excess salt consumption, the circumstantial evidence is pretty convincing. If you must use canned baby food, select low-sodium varieties and protect the health of your child.

There is little point in torturing the family's taste buds by leaving salt out of your cooking. Most of our excess sodium comes hidden in processed foods. Table 5 gives you some examples of items that may not taste terribly salty but in fact have huge amounts of added sodium. These are compared with fresh foods. To preserve your health, keep salt intake to 1,000 mg (half a small teaspoon) a day. Salt is useful for melting snow on sidewalks. That's where it should stay, firmly underfoot.

We Eat More Hidden Sugar Every Year

It's a pity sugar does not melt snow. Processed food is stuffed with this terrible sweetener, for which there seems to be no safe

Table 5: Sodium Content of Fresh and Processed Foods (mg sodium per 100 g [3½ oz])

Fresh Food	*Sodium*	*Processed Food*	*Sodium*
Beefsteak	60	Bologna	1,300
Pork loin	290	Frankfurter	1,100
Chicken	50	Bacon	680
Sockeye salmon	48	Canned salmon	520
Flounder, sole	80	Sardines in tomato sauce	400
Oysters	73	Canned oysters	206
Cabbage	20	Sauerkraut	750
Asparagus	2	Canned asparagus	240
Tomatoes	3	Tomato ketchup	1,040
Peas	1	Canned peas	230
Peanuts	5	Peanut butter	600
Potatoes	3	Potato chips	1,000
Onions	10	Pickled onions	1,420
Homemade vegetable soup with salt to taste	60	Canned vegetable soup	400
Plain popcorn	3	Salted popcorn	1,940
Whole wheat flour	2	Graham crackers	670
White flour	2	Pretzels	1,680
Wheat germ	3	Self-rising flour	1,080
White or brown rice	9	Puffed rice cereal	360
Whole cow's milk	50	Cheddar cheese	700
Human milk	16	Canned baby food	300

(See Reference 16)

alternative. With most of our food now processed, we get an enormous sugar overload. This does not count obvious sources such as hard candy, chocolate and ice cream. They would remain fine treats if we were not burdened with sugar hidden elsewhere. The average American diet is now 20 percent refined sugar, half a pound a day per person.[33] Even frozen turkeys now have sugar added. The effects of sugar in producing the current epidemics of obesity, diabetes and heart disease are well documented in the chapters on these maladies.

The tendency to like sweet substances probably developed

during evolution as an adaptive mechanism to ensure that the human species ate the plants in which sugars occur, plants which also contain most of the vitamins and minerals needed for health. Our recent sweet-sick syndrome is a result of technological developments which permit extraction of the sugars from their nutritious context. So we still have the inherited urge to eat sweets, but most of the sweets we are offered to eat are nutritionally valueless.

Worse, just like refined flour, the major fault of refined sugar is that *it no longer contains the nutrients required for its own metabolism.*[34] In order to digest refined sugar and use it, the body has to rob itself by consuming its own supplies of B vitamins. Considering the deficiencies of B vitamins in the American diet discussed earlier in this chapter, ingestion of excess sugar is therefore the likely basis of much degenerative disease.

We are not often told this, because sugar is *very* profitable. In coming out against it nutritionally in 1979, the Surgeon General courageously attacked one of the most powerful lobbies in the country.[35] Tame scientists retained by the sugar industry are continually telling us that sugar is harmless. Our inherited liking for sweets continually makes us want to believe them. For most of us the only answer lies in avoiding hidden sugar. Products often touted as healthy, or at least harmless, are some of the worst offenders. A large glass of cola (12 oz), for example, contains seven teaspoons of sugar (1½ oz). The same amount of cream soda or fruit-flavored sodas contains nearer 2 oz of sugar. With their added caffeine as well, soft drinks must rank as *the* most unhealthy food product on the market. Yet because of clever promotion, our per capita consumption of these beverages rises year after year.

Other foods that have more hidden sugar than commonly thought are breakfast cereals. Some of the Kellogg products, such as Apple Jacks and Sugar Snacks, are more than half sugar. Giving your child a chocolate bar and a glass of milk for breakfast would be just as nutritious. Some others are low in sugar but high in sodium, up to 700 mg per 4-oz serving. Unfortunately, the names of cereals are forever being changed to catch the "novelty" share of the market, so it is difficult to keep track of the worst ones. Best to avoid the habit of eating refined cereals at all. As with refined sugar, in being digested they steal more of the body's nutrients than they contain.[36] Like refined sugar also, they provide only empty calories, calories that have made America one of the fattest nations on earth.

Other hidden sources of sugar are the so-called health foods. Most of the bars and candies in health-food stores are loaded with disguised sugar. We examined seventy-two different brands and found only two without sugar. And those two tasted—yech! Terms used to disguise the sugar content range through turbinado sugar, grape sugar, date sugar, corn syrup, galactose, fructose, dextrose, levulose, maltose and others never seen in a dictionary. Some manufacturers of "health food" candy use several different sugars, so they can list them further down the contents list. Then sugar doesn't look like a major ingredient. Added together, these sugars may be *the* major ingredient. Even carob is 50 percent sugar. The only advantage of carob over chocolate is absence of caffeine. When you just have to indulge your inherited sweet tooth, don't fool yourself with "health food" candy. Might as well really enjoy yourself with a triple mint-chip and chocolate sauce.

Not many of us could become saints of the Pritikin program and give up all our sugars. Fortunately, such a sacrifice isn't necessary. Our work with obese patients and lean athletes led to a delightful discovery concerning sugar and refined flours. We were studying the effects of individually designed vitamin and mineral supplements and eating patterns on controlling the urge to binge. Binging on cakes and candy produces not only obesity and vitamin deficiency, but also metabolic, circulatory and cardiac abnormalities.[37] We monitored these variables and discovered that it required up to seventy-two hours for all these measures to return to normal. So, in order to participate, the fatties and the athletes used as controls had to restrict processed sugars, starches and the processed fats in these foods for three days before they were allowed a one-day binge. Then they avoided all processed foods for another three days after all their physiological functions had returned to normal. So, the binge-restrict cycle was seven days long. All of these people ate far more calories on the binge than they had cut out of their diets during the restricted period. Yet they *consistently lost weight.* Even the athletes lost three to five pounds in the four weeks of the study, although they were very lean to begin with. The main reason for these results is that the body has a limited capacity to digest sugars and starches at any one time. If you spread your extra carbohydrates out over the week, however, it will grab all of them.

After the study ended, most of the patients adopted the strategy of allowing themselves one binge a week, and we adopted the strategy of advising all obese patients to do it. In combination with the other weight-reducing strategies described in Chapter 8, this tactic has helped some patients to control their weight very successfully for more than six years. The individually designed vitamin and mineral supplements reduce the urge to eat, and the weekly binge seems to offset the feelings of martyrdom and malaise that cause most diets to fail. In the words of one now-trim lady, "Before I came to you, I had been dieting for twenty-seven years and was gradually losing the battle. Now, I can eat like a mouse all week, because Saturday I munch to paradise. Saturday is sin day."

Our specially designed vitamin and mineral supplements probably inhibit the craving for food in several ways. First, because they are designed for each individual, they eliminate the specific hungers that result from particular deficiencies. A well-known example is the unsupplemented mother's craving for strange edibles during pregnancy, triggered by the huge nutrient needs of the growing fetus, especially the needs for folic acid and calcium. The craving may be translated into demands for entirely the wrong kind of food, leaving the mother unsatisfied, wanting something else but not sure what. Correct supplementation completely eliminates this craving. Second, the supplements stabilize blood-sugar levels, reducing the sugar-dependent hunger common in the overweight. Third, the supplements eliminate the nonspecific syndrome of anxiety, fatigue, muscle and joint pain, insomnia, irregularity and depression evident in 80 percent of people we have tested who eat a lot of processed food.[38] Of course, you don't have to be overweight to get these benefits from the supplements. They have the same effects for anyone who lives on the myth of the good mixed diet.

CHAPTER 3

PRINCIPLES OF VITAMIN/MINERAL SUPPLEMENTATION

FOR MANY PEOPLE the annual physical is their main attempt at preventive medicine. In the guise of prevention, these checkups have given people a false sense of security about their health. Physicals are not preventive at all—they can only *detect* disease *after* it is established.[1] Because medicine itself developed out of the study of infectious diseases, physicians are trained to pursue the pathological, that is, sickness. Most doctors know nothing about how to prevent a disease before it shows any symptoms. How doctors are confined by their training to detective disease hunts was illustrated recently in an examination of some of our patients successfully treated with vitamin supplements. The excellent physician doing the tests exclaimed, "Give me time. I'll find *something wrong* with them." It is a sad criticism of medicine that he had no means of looking for *something right.*

Detective physical examinations are doubly bad. Not only do they fail to prevent disease, they also fail to detect it. For example, an extensive study done for the Kaiser Health Plan in California tested ten thousand people between ages thirty-five and fifty-four. Five thousand of them were given frequent medical examinations and five thousand were not. Over seven years there was no difference between the groups in the incidence of disease, in the incidence of disability or in death rate.[2] In another study, in Baltimore, Dr. Lewis Kuller found that 326 people who died of sudden heart attacks in one year had been medically examined within the preceding six months, 86 within seven days before death. Not a single death had been predicted by their doctors.[3] Another study examined the deaths of 350 executives who had regular, intensive health examinations. In almost half the deaths the fatal disease had not been detected beforehand.[4]

Many other investigations have produced similar findings,[5] but the most comprehensive evidence is the 1979 report of the Canadian Task Force on the Periodic Health Examination.[6] This extensive, three-year study concluded that annual physical examinations are ineffective and should be discarded. The report recommended instead that health-protection packages be developed for groups in high-risk categories. These recommendations have yet to be implemented. Until they are, which will be in 1995 at the earliest, you must protect yourself.

Does Your Physician Know About Nutrition?

Your physician cannot help you prevent vitamin and mineral deficiencies, because he probably knows very little about nutrition. This is a serious charge, especially when the Surgeon General lists faulty nutrition as one of the six causes of America's burden of degenerative disease.[7] So I had better give you good evidence that medical training has failed to keep up with the science of nutrition.

One pertinent proof of modern medicine's failure in the nutritional field is the hospital malnutrition discussed in the last chapter. Every hospital study undertaken has found serious malnutrition among patients. The latest studies have shown that the patients became malnourished *after* admission to the hospital, and *not* because of their illness but as a direct result of the nutritionally deficient diet provided.[8] In 1980 Dr. Maurice Shils, director of Clinical Nutrition at Sloan-Kettering Hospital in New York, deplored the ignorance of many physicians when confronted with hospital malnutrition.[9] If doctors cannot prevent malnutrition with all the facilities of a hospital at hand, you cannot expect them to help you prevent it.

The problem first loomed in the 1960's, when modern nutrition science began to accelerate. In 1964 Dr. W. H. Sebrell of Columbia University showed that medical education in nutrition was lagging far behind advances in nutrition science.[10] In 1968 Professor Frederick Stare, head of Harvard's Department of Nutrition, described how bad medical education in nutrition was.[11] In 1969 the White House Conference on Food, Nutrition and Health concluded that "the teaching of nutrition in schools of medicine, dentistry and nursing is most inadequate at the present time."[12] In 1971 the *American Journal of Clinical Nutrition* showed that doctors get virtually no training in applied nutrition.[13] Dr. Julian Schorr of the New York Blood Center put it aptly: "Often doctors are trained in nutrition by doctors who heard it from another doctor who made it up."[14] In 1972 Dr. Michael Latham of Cornell concluded that "nine out of ten doctors in New York would give wrong answers to dietary questions."[15] In 1976 the Department of Health, Education and Welfare emphasized the abundant evidence that current medical detection and treatment services do not favorably influence the health of the nation.[16] Enough said!

There is a growing association of excellent young physicians and some pioneering, vigorous oldsters who are correcting this deficit. Through extra study and training they have educated themselves in nutrition and prevention of disease. These new doctors, all fine examples of their own prescriptions, will eventually take over. The more that you, the public, who pay for all medicine, demand doctors who are knowledgeable about nutrition and prevention of disease, the quicker they will become the norm. If you are ill, you can find one of these physicians in your home area by writing to: The Huxley Institute, 1114 First Avenue, New York, NY 10021.

The need for such training has finally struck home at the official level too, partly through the admirable emphasis on prevention by Secretary of Health Richard Schweiker. In 1981 the American Board of Nutrition began arranging for recognition of clinical nutrition as a medical specialty, and called for assistance from university researchers in nutrition to define goals and standards.[17] Unfortunately, the first nutrition-oriented doctors to result from this laudable action will not be seen before 1990 at the earliest. Meanwhile, you must learn to protect yourself. To do so, you need to appreciate how nature made you to function optimally only if you have a continual supply of a unique blend of nutrients.

Evolution Controls the Mixture

Evolution developed our bodies to use the multiple interactions of certain substances that occur in nature. The composition of your blood serum is almost identical to the composition of the seawater from which our reptilian ancestors once crawled for short, uncomfortable sojourns on land. Now, we carry our ocean around inside us. In fact, the hairy bags of salty soup we call human beings ARE the multiple interactions of some basic simple chemicals. The mystery and wonder of human life is how our genes, our genesis, came to lay down a plan that can turn inert chemicals into collections of living human cells capable of love, joy, courage and myriad emotions. Most of all, capable of the determination to understand their own nature and purpose.

To date, seventeen vitamins and cofactors (that is, helper substances), eight amino acids (ten for children and some adults) and twenty-four minerals are recognized as essential to the human genetic plan.[18] These are listed in Table 6. A few of the substances listed, such as arsenic and tin, are present in so many foods and are required in such minute amounts that they are provided in some measure by all diets. It is very difficult to eliminate them so as to demonstrate a clear deficiency in humans, because even these tiny specks must be absent for periods of up to one hundred days for deficiency symptoms to

Table 6: Essential Elements and Micronutrients (Substances that may be deficient in the American diet are shown in bold type)

Elements Required in Large Amounts Daily			
hydrogen (H)	carbon (C)	nitrogen (N)	oxygen (O)
sulfur (S)			
Elements Required in Medium Amounts Daily			
calcium (Ca)	**magnesium (Mg)**	phosphorus (P)	**potassium (K)**
sodium (Na)	chlorine (Cl)		
Elements Required in Small Amounts Daily			
iron (Fe)	**iodine (I)**	**manganese (Mn)**	**zinc (Zn)**
vanadium (V)	**chromium (Cr)**	**cobalt (Co)**	nickel (Ni)
molybdenum (Mo)	**selenium (Se)**	fluorine (F)	
copper (Cu)	silicon (Si)	tin (Sn)*	arsenic (As)*
* probable essential minerals			
Vitamins and Cofactors (common-form names)			
A (retinol)	**C (ascorbic acid)**	bioflavonoids	**D (calciferol)**
E (d-alpha-tocopherol)		K (menadione)	
B_1 (thiamine)	**B_2 (riboflavin)**	**B_3 (niacin)**	**B_5 (pantothenic acid)**
B_6 (pyridoxine)	**B_{12} (cobalamin)**	**folic acid**	para-amino-benzoic acid (PABA)
choline	inositol	**biotin**	
Essential Amino Acids			
isoleucine	leucine	**lysine**	**methionine**
phenylalanine	threonine	tryptophan	valine
arginine (children)		histidine (children)	

Eight criteria were used to determine probable deficiencies: nutrient content of foods, dominant dietary habits, degrees of bioavailability, ranges of individual requirements, additional nutritional demands of American lifestyle, and additional nutritional demands caused by deliberate bodily pollution and unavoidable bodily pollution.

show. Animals, however, can be confined and fed super-pure diets lacking only the particular mineral under study. When deficiency has been shown in several species, as it has for all substances listed in Table 6, it is a good bet that the nutrient is required for human health too.

Two aspects of this list require special note. First, many of the substances were established as essential only in the last fifteen years. Consequently, practicing physicians trained before 1965 may know nothing about them. For example, prior to 1965 chromium was thought to be more appropriate for car bumpers than human bodies. Now, we know that chromium deficiency causes glucose intolerance. We know also that this disorder can be corrected by supplemental chromium.[19]

Second, we are certain the list is incomplete. Many elements and other substances are now under intense study. Tin was not shown to be essential to animal growth until 1970,[20] and still waits to be proved essential to human health. Arsenic has been used as a growth stimulant in pigs and poultry for decades,[21] but not until 1975 was it reported to be *essential* for animal health.[22] It is probably required for human health too. *But don't take any.* You get ample arsenic in your diet. Though it has taken science the last hundred years to do so, knowing which nutrients are essential is the easy part. The hard part is finding out what happens to them once they get inside you.

Nutrients Operate by Multiple Interactions

Only recently has medical science accepted how tightly the human body and nature are interlocked. The surge of twentieth-century technology deluded us into thinking we could capture nature in a test tube. Now, we know, humbly, that we cannot. The human test tube is quite different from the laboratory flask. Prior to 1970 many silly experiments were done with single vitamins and minerals *in vitro* (in the test tube) on which many silly recommendations were made for human nutrition. Now, we know there is *never* a deficiency of just one vitamin or mineral. There is *never* any vitamin or mineral activity by itself. The multiple interactions of these essential substances is the basis of their biological function. And the adequacy of that function depends on the substances being supplied to the body in the same mixtures and concentrations that occur in raw, unprocessed foods. It was by use of these foods that genesis, over millions of years of evolution, developed the precise mechanisms to deal with them.

Controversy is rife over the use of vitamins, mainly because scientists have relied on evidence from single-nutrient studies. Many single-nutrient studies have failed to show effects because complementary nutrients were not sufficiently available in the diet. Single-nutrient studies on humans *never* give single-nutrient results. Vitamin C to stop colds, for example, depends as much on other nutrients in the diet as on the supplemental Vitamin C. If the diet is deficient in nutrients which interact with Vitamin C in promoting resistance to colds, it is impossible for the body to use the C supplement. The *minimum* of supplementary nutrients required are adequate B_6 (pyridoxine), B_{12} (cobalamin), zinc, folic acid and choline.[23]

Such interdependent interactions as that between calcium and Vitamin D have been known for a long time. But we have established only recently *that every nutrient and essential element operates by multiple interactions.* For example, a deficiency of Vitamin A, apart from its well-known effects on the skin and eyes, leads to abnormal metabolism of iron, resulting in anemia.[24] Vitamin A deficiency also reduces calcium metabolism, resulting in poor bone growth.[25] Moreover, a Vitamin A deficiency can occur even when the diet is adequately supplying the nutrient; Vitamin A becomes deficient in the tissue as a result of dietary deficiency of zinc, one of the minerals on which Vitamin A is dependent for its proper utilization by the body.[26] Alcoholics frequently have low serum A and resultant night blindness.

Often they cannot be helped by the use of Vitamin A supplements alone, but addition of zinc normalizes both serum A and night vision.[27]

Take one more example of multiple interactions. Pellagra used to be thought of as simply a B_3-deficiency disease. You need less than 20 mg of B_3 a day to prevent "the 3D syndrome" of pellagra: diarrhea, dermatitis, dementia. But we know that the clinical symptoms which occur long before obvious pellagra are caused by multiple vitamin deficiencies. In the early 1970's, when we began this work, children were often referred to our clinics for "psychosomatic" disorders. Some of them showed gastrointestinal disturbances, loss of appetite and intermittent diarrhea, and the "beef-red, shiny tongue syndrome" characteristic of incipient pellagra. The symptoms did not seem to get worse with time. Nor did they respond to a B_3 supplement. So, intitially we thought we were wrong, and pellagra was not involved. We quickly learned better. Now, we know that well before the pellagra appears, B_2, B_6 and the amino acid tryptophan are also likely to be deficient, in addition to B_3.[28] In turn, these deficiencies affect other nutrients. B_2 deficiency impairs B_{12} metabolism, threatening to cause anemia. B_6 deficiency impairs C metabolism, which in turn impairs folic-acid metabolism.[29] The resultant depletion of the body's Vitamin C impairs iron absorption.[30] Impaired iron absorption, combined with low dietary iron, encourages excessive copper absorption, which in turn interferes with zinc metabolism,[31] creating a danger of jaundice. Excess copper also affects nickel metabolism, which further affects iron metabolism,[32] and on and on and on. In the case of the nutritionally deficient children brought to our clinic, nothing short of a complete vitamin and mineral supplement which permitted all these essential interactions to occur normally sufficed to bring these youngsters back to good health.

Long ago we abandoned any use of the classical vitamin-deficiency syndromes and their traditional treatment. Yet the RDAs are still based upon these outmoded concepts. Now, when medical science knows of the thousands of multiple, interdependent interactions of nutrients and mineral elements that are essential to good health, citing the RDAs as a basis for human nutrition is absurd. It is the medical focus on disease rather than on prevention that has kept us in this muddle. When we focus instead on prevention, the need for a complete and balanced blend of all essential nutrients immediately becomes apparent.

Biochemical Individuality Lays the Ground Plan

You are biologically unique. In size, weight, shape, position and function, your muscles, glands, nerves, organs and brain are like no one else's on earth. From where your hair grows to the speed with which your blood flows, your body plays a unique symphony. We all accept the uniqueness of fingerprints. We all respond to an unmistakably familiar voice, unique because of the exclusive shape and function of each individual's mouth, throat and larynx. But many people do not realize that every part of their body differs radically from the form and function described in standard anatomy textbooks. Your perfectly normal stomach may have two chambers instead of the textbook one.[33] And the digestive juices your stomach uses may be a hundred times stronger, or weaker, than the next person's. Compared to the mythical textbook average, you may have inherited a fast or slow brain, low or high blood pressure, poor or keen eyesight, sharp or dull hearing, high or low sex hormones, sluggish or explosive thyroid, and a zillion other variations. The unique combinations are endless. And they require unique fuel. For optimum health you need a blend of nutrients different from anyone else's. This *biochemical individuality* is the second principle of effective supplementation.

In the 1920's renowned physiologist Carl Lashley found that there were so many variations in body structure and function between different members of the same species *that they were more like different species.* Since then, over many years Professor Roger Williams has patiently documented thousands of differences in function between individuals, including many differences in individual needs for nutrients.[34] In animals, for example, he found that some rats seem to need forty times as much Vitamin A as others.[35] For optimum growth some guinea pigs required twenty times as much Vitamin C as others.[36]

In my clinic and laboratory we routinely measure Vitamin C excretion in the urine of patients and athletes. At first we were trying to find out whether supplemental Vitamin C is simply excreted from the human body, so that all you get from taking Vitamin C is expensive urine, as some medical scientists have claimed. We showed that they are dead wrong. Some people could take 5,000 mg of Vitamin C and excrete almost none at all. All that Vitamin C was being used by their bodies in the hundreds of biological functions Vitamin C is known to have.[37] Other people did excrete increased Vitamin C, but only a fraction of the amount swallowed. We found the range of usage in different people to be tenfold.

The expensive urine argument is wrong in any case. Excretion of vitamins and minerals is part of the normal functioning of the body. You do it every day. If you stop doing it, then something has gone haywire. You excrete your urine and feces because they are poisonous to the body. The body is designed to ensure that its excretions contain vitamins and minerals so as to protect the intestines, bowels and urinary tract from damage by its own toxic wastes. Because of the high levels of both deliberate and unavoidable bodily pollution today, our body wastes are highly toxic; an excellent reason for ensuring that we keep daily excretion of protective vitamins and minerals at a high level. Expensive? No. A bargain. The average victim of bowel or bladder cancer spends twenty-six thousand dollars for treatment—mostly to no avail.

We measured how much Vitamin C the body can use by giving graduated amounts over a ten-week period. We started with 500 mg a day the first week, on weekdays only. Then we increased the daily supplement by 500 mg each week to a maximum of 5,000 mg a day. On the Monday, after a Saturday and Sunday with no Vitamin C, we took fasting urine samples before the subjects took their Vitamin C, and again five to six hours afterward (with no intervening urination). When the urine showed increased excretion of Vitamin C (by a certain percentage above the fasting level), that was taken as the maximum the body could use. The results are shown in Figure 1. Only a quarter of our subjects reached their Vitamin C maximum at a level of 1,500 mg a day. More than half of them required over 2,500 mg a day to reach a level where their bodies could use no more. Four subjects did not reach their maximum at 5,000 mg.

This huge variation in the amount of Vitamin C required to reach what is called tissue-saturation level indicates a biochemical individuality that makes nonsense of any determination of an average requirement. We read of the average family size being 2.4 children. Yet we do not start looking for 0.4 of a child. We know 2.4 is a statistical average, and families may vary from 1 to 18 children. Yet when we are told that the average amount of Vitamin C required is 60 mg a day, somehow this number takes on a sacred significance. It is time scientists, nutritionists and food manufacturers stopped all the silliness about the RDAs. They have nothing to do with the nutritional status of an individual. They are intended for use in estimating the adequacy of food supplies for the whole population as a unit, in order to prevent the occurrence of certain deficiency diseases.[38] From my own work, and the work of Dr. Sherry Lewin in Britain,[39] and of Drs. Linus Pauling, Brian Leibovitz and Benjamin Siegel in America,[40] among many others, the amount of Vitamin C required to prevent scurvy, the basis of the RDA, bears no relation to the widely varying amounts of Vitamin C required by different individuals for optimum health.

Just to mention the hundreds of papers showing biochemical individuality for other nutrients would more than fill the rest of this book. Individual needs for amino acids,[41] vitamins[42] and minerals[43] are amply documented. I will give only one more example. Medical science is making rapid progress concerning

***Figure 1:** Maximum amounts of daily Vitamin C absorbed (5 percent of subjects did not reach maximum at 5.0 grams. 1 percent of subjects were excluded for noncompliance.) Maximum calculated from a variable percentage increase (depending on dosage) in excreted repeated urine samples using dichlorophenolindophenol*

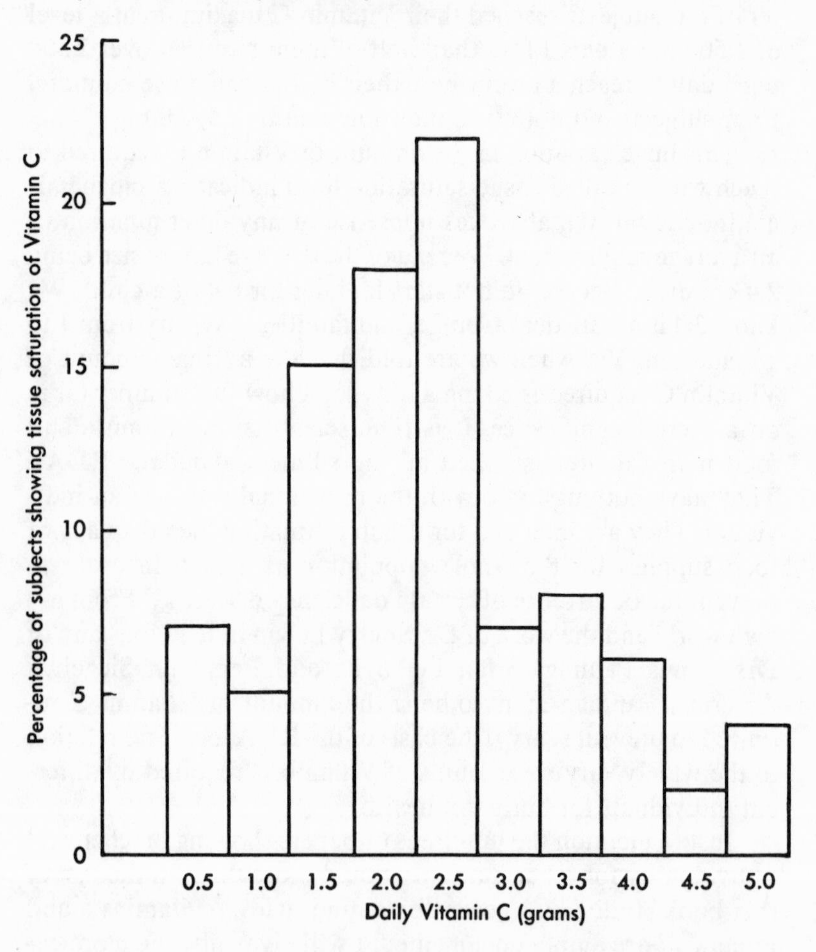

what is called the major histocompatibility complex and the immune system, the principal defenses of the body against disease and degeneration. Simply put, the histocompatibility complex is your body's unique identity code, given to you by your genes. It is a series of structures in the membranes of your cells by which the body recognizes its own cells and kills or rejects foreign cells or substances. The precise action of your body's histocompatibility complex is different from anyone else's on earth and requires unique nutritional support for optimum function. Whenever your nutrition is faulty, or you are poisoned by drugs or other nonbiological pollutants, your immune system's unique capacity to recognize and deal with foreign cells is weakened.[44]

Aging and degenerative disease are a progressive failure of the body to protect its identity. More and more foreign cells and substances take up residence, leading inevitably to degeneration. In the next chapter we will consider the abundant new evidence that vitamin supplementation improves the operation of the immune system.[45] When the immune system is working optimally, it is impossible for foreign cells, bacteria, viruses or poisons to remain in the body. In December 1980, as he received the Nobel Prize for his work on the histocompatibility complex, Dr. Jean Dausset said:

> An inventory of the immunological capacities of each individual will need to be drawn up. . . . In this way, preventive medicine of high precision will be possible; a personalized medicine that will be more efficient and less burdensome for the community than the present mass system.[46]

By using the principle of biochemical individuality *now* to design your own nutrition, you are stealing a march on the preventive medicine of the twenty-first century.

Lifestyle and Dietary Habits Determine the Amounts

It would be easy to design individual supplements if heredity alone determined your individual needs for nutrients. Unfortunately, what you and your environment do to your body radically affects your needs also. Nutritional requirements vary with diet, smoking, alcohol, pollution, contraception, pregnancy, medication, occupation, exercise, age and many other variables. In our clinics the assessment instruction manual runs to three volumes just to cover the possibilities we know about. We add new ones every week. As many of these variables as possible have been incorporated into the self-assessment system detailed in Chapter 6.

Diet determines in large part the need for supplemental nutrients. We have seen already that the average diet can be a life sentence of degenerative disease—with refined sugar and processed carbohydrate that pull nutrients from the body, with excess salt, with denatured bread and with fruit and vegetables that have lost most of their nutrients. No wonder government studies have found widespread nutritional deficiencies in America today. Although the various studies measured only twelve of the thirty-one nutrients likely to be deficient (see Table 6), and took these measurements using the conservative RDA standards, widespread deficiencies were found in nine of them: vitamins A, B_1, B_2, B_6, C, folic acid and minerals iron, calcium and magnesium.

Endemic goiter exemplifies how insufficiency of even a single essential nutrient can result in widespread degenerative disease. When the daily diet lacks 1/10,000 of a gram of iodine (too small to see), thyroid function is disrupted, and consequently many other bodily processes. The most serious complication of iodine deficiency is the type of mental retardation called cretinism. The prominent visible sign is a swelling of the thyroid gland that straddles the windpipe in the small hollow where the neck joins the chest. It used to be so common in the "Goiter Belt" of middle America, where there is insufficient iodine in the soil, that the swelling of incipient goiter filling the hollow was considered a beauty mark of the full flower of American womanhood.

Iodizing our table salt (*a simple preventive measure*) markedly reduced the incidence of obvious goiter. But incipient goiter still occurs frequently. Hypothyroidism, a related condition also associated with iodine deficiency, is extremely prevalent. Together, the two are estimated to affect a staggering *90 million* Americans.[47] Hence the widespread use of synthetic thyroid hormones for all sorts of nonspecific complaints.

Two dietary causes are involved in this epidemic thyroid malfunction. First, many people have wisely restricted their use of table salt in an attempt to prevent hypertension. In doing so, however, they inadvertently restrict their iodine. Second, vegetables of the genus *Brassica,* including Brussels sprouts, cabbage, kale, mustard, rutabaga, turnips and watercress, contain compounds called thioglucosides, which disrupt thyroid function. Their effect is blocked only if there is ample iodine in the diet.[48] Drugs such as the sulphonamides, used routinely for urinary tract infections, also interfere with iodine metabolism and disrupt thyroid function. These factors and many others are taken into account in calculating your nutrient needs.

The need for Vitamin B_6 is also greatly influenced by diet. All diets high in saturated fats, that is, all diets including regular bacon, ham, steak, butter, cheese and fried foods, may increase the need for B_6 as much as fivefold,[49] because B_6 is used in maintaining normal fat metabolism.[50] If you eat a lot of preserved meats—bologna, sausage, wursts, bacon—you will need more than B_6 to protect you. Most processed meats contain deliberately added nitrates and nitrites as preservatives and color-enhancers. These additives prevent the growth of deadly botulism bacteria in these products. Unfortunately, nitrates and nitrites form carcinogenic nitrosamines, both in cooking and in interaction with digestive juices. Today some manufacturers add the antioxidant Vitamin C to sausages and bacon, which blocks formation of nitrosamines. This is not a satisfactory answer, however. Nitrosamines form in the human digestive tract in what are called the aqueous, lipid and micellar stages of digestion, roughly speaking, in the watery, oily and fatty stages. Vitamin C, being water-soluble only, acts only in the watery phase.

The fat-soluble Vitamin E is needed to block nitrosamine formation in the other two phases.[51] So, people who like their knackwurst require not only ample B_6 for the fat metabolism, but also ample amounts of C and E to protect themselves against the nitrate threat of cancer.

Eating the Nutrients Is No Guarantee

You have seen what is lost in the cooking. Now see what is lost in the eating. The bioavailability of nutrients is greatly influenced by your diet. One example is the essential mineral zinc, which is already 25 percent deficient in the American diet,[52] even taking the RDA of 15 mg per day as an adequate standard. The RDA allows for 3 mg to be bioavailable, that is, to be successfully extracted from the food by digestion and absorbed undamaged for use by the body. *On the average* 3 mg will suffice for bodily needs. By normal digestive processes the rest is destroyed, excreted or bound with other substances so that it is unavailable. The typical American diet, however, contains lots of cereals, with milk and breads as staple foods. All breads and cereals contain compounds called phytates which bind with zinc and prevent the body from using it. Whenever milk is taken also, the calcium serves to increase this binding action. Such a diet can reduce the bioavailable zinc to less than 1 mg per 15 mg of zinc in the food.[53] To get the 3 mg necessary for the average person, at least an additional 30 mg of zinc is required, making 45 mg in all. When we know that zinc in the average American diet is below the RDA already (average 11–12 mg), severe zinc deficiency resulting directly from dietary habits is very likely. The catalogue of illnesses that may result has been ably documented by Dr. Carl Pfeiffer.[54] It includes dwarfism, liver disease, impotence, diabetes, mental disorder and cancer, making zinc deficiency a condition we should carefully avoid.

Anemias from dietary deficiencies of iron and folic acid are so widespread in America that we tend to consider them as normal. Like zinc deficiency, anemias depend not only on the nutrients in the food but also on our dietary habits. Studies by world expert Dr. Virgil Fairbanks and his colleagues have now shown that almost all pregnant women are iron deficient.[55] One in every two American women is likely to be iron deficient *all her adult life.*[56] Iron in the American diet is insufficient for all women from their teenage years on.[57] Those who avoid meat in an attempt to lower fat intake to prevent cardiovascular disease are especially at risk, because only about 3 percent of the iron in vegetables is bioavailable. Overall, 10 percent of the iron in food is bioavailable. If your diet contains regular eggs, tea or bran cereals, however, you may get less than 5 percent, because these foods inhibit iron absorption.

Simple supplementation with iron is not the answer, however, because of absorption limits and side-effect problems, notably stomach pain, nausea and constipation. With iron supplements alone, it can take six months to replenish iron stores after pregnancy.[58] Vitamin C enhances iron absorption, but the huge number of interactions of iron with other nutrients indicates that a complete nutrient supplement is the best answer.

Folic acid is deficient in about one third of pregnant women, even in many who are taking folic-acid supplements.[59] It may be that the widespread deficiencies of the B vitamins (discussed in Chapter 2) which operate in synergy with folic acid are preventing proper absorption and utilization of this nutrient. Unlike iron, folic acid is easy to obtain in the diet by eating *raw* fruits and vegetables daily. The existence of widespread folate deficiency, together with widespread Vitamin A deficiency, shows that *we simply do not eat our greens.* Unfortunately, a desirable change in our eating habits is highly unlikely when the USDA, the official guardian of our nutrition, sets such a bad example in trying to classify ketchup as a school-lunch vegetable.

Deliberate Pollution: The Weed and the Bottle

Thanks to the Surgeon General, most of us now know that smoking causes cancers, cardiovascular disease, bronchitis, emphysema, peptic ulcers and the low birth-weight syndrome.[60] The effects of smoking on nutrition are involved in all these diseases. Many people don't yet realize that medical experts concluded in 1981 that there is no safe level of smoking. Attempts to make a safe cigarette have failed.[61] Worse, if someone consistently smokes near you indoors, your disease risk can be that of a ten-cigarettes-a-day smoker.[62] So even if you don't smoke, other people smoking around you are depleting the nutrients in *your* body.

Let's look at just one of tobacco's many effects. Smoking suppresses the immune system by destroying the Vitamin C required by the leucocytes (white cells), one of the body's main defenders against disease.[63] As we saw in Chapter 2, we are already deficient in Vitamin C even without smoking. The HANES survey in 1972 concluded that more than a third of Americans have insufficient Vitamin C in their diets, even at the inadequate RDA standard of 60 mg a day.[64] So, smokers and their hapless companions are doubly deprived. Fortunately, Vitamin C supplementation quickly restores immune-system function.[65] Everyone exposed to smoking has an increased requirement for Vitamin C.

Alcohol puts quite different nutritional demands on the body. These demands are so diverse and complex that scientists will be busily engaged for many more years just to define them. We do know that more than three drinks a day (1½ oz alcohol) leads to slow liver degeneration and increased risk of cancer, cardiovascular disease and mental disorder.[66] Reliable estimates indicate that one person in five drinks too much.[67] That's fifty million Americans! The confirmed alcoholics, totaling seventeen million, have multiple vitamin and mineral deficiencies, including A, B_3, B_6, C, magnesium, zinc and essential fatty acids.[68]

The same nutrients are probably deficient in moderate drinkers. The best evidence that even a moderate consumption of alcohol may damage your nutrition is the fetal alcohol syndrome. The infant born to a mother taking even two drinks a day (1 oz alcohol) may have facial-shape abnormalities, low birth weight and mental retardation.[69] Coupled with the poor maternal nutrition described earlier, drinking during pregnancy is a double no-no. Each year, more than one hundred thousand babies are born mentally retarded from various causes. A large proportion of these human tragedies are alcohol-related. Your best bet is not to drink at all during pregnancy. After weaning, however, occasional indulgence will not hurt you. It is regular alcohol abuse that produces degenerative disease. Your body can easily deal with an occasional binge.

Unavoidable Pollution Also Destroys Nutrients

Even if you eat perfectly and have no vices, you cannot avoid exposure to toxic metals and other substances which build up in your body to destroy your health. These toxic pollutants include cadmium from cigarette smoke and polluted fish; aluminum from antacids, toothpastes, shampoos, deodorants and cookware; mercury from hair dyes, petroleum products, agricultural uses, fish and cosmetics; and lead from leaded gasoline, cosmetics, fertilizers and canned foods. We are also exposed to sulfur and nitrogen oxides, insecticides like Kepone, plasticizers like polychlorinated biphenyls (PCBs) and carcinogenic plastics like polyvinyl chlorides (PVCs). The list is endless. In 1979 the Surgeon General indicted the hundreds of toxic pollutants in the American environment as major causes of degenerative disease.[70] Many of the precise effects of these pollutants are unknown. Our only defense is to keep bodily resistance as high as possible with optimum nutrition, because *all* the pollutants we do know about deplete the body of nutrients.

The poisonous metal cadmium attacks people deficient in any of the following—Vitamins C, D, B_6, zinc, iron, manganese, copper, selenium or calcium.[71] All people in urban areas need ample stores of these nutrients, because cadmium inhibits their normal function. Urban cadmium pollution is now at 50 mcg per person per day, a level that threatens to cause kidney and adrenal damage and anemia.[72] Cadmium builds up silently and slowly in the kidneys and the liver over many years, because once in, very little is excreted from the body.[73] It was once thought that nothing could remove cadmium deposits. Now, thankfully, superb scientific detective work has shown that iron and Vitamin C together reduce body cadmium,[74] and an ample intake of selenium and zinc is the best protection against cadmium toxicity.[75]

Aluminum is a prevalent pollutant too. It is involved in many diseases, including Alzheimer's insanity.[76] Another evil of aluminum pollution is that it inhibits fluorine and phosphorus metabolism, resulting over a long period of time in a loss of minerals from the bones and consequent osteoporosis (fragile bones).[77] In November 1981 *The Harvard Medical School Newsletter* stated that America is experiencing an epidemic of osteoporosis in the elderly. The disease begins thirty years before any symptoms appear. The seed is sown at about age thirty-five. Aluminum is not the only factor, but it provides an excellent example of the "action at a distance" of bodily pollution in producing degenerative disease. To avoid aluminum pollution, do not use on or in your body any product that has "alumina," "aluminate," "aluminum" or similar words on its contents list. Also, ditch those aluminum pots and pans.

The level of mercury pollution in American bodies causes few cases of clear-cut disease. Common signs of mercury pollution are nonspecific depression, irritability, tremor, dizziness and diarrhea. But as the metal builds up over a number of years, it leads to progressive degeneration of the brain, liver, kidneys and intestines, finally causing the "Mad Hatter" syndrome, the insanity that used to be common among milliners and furriers, as a consequence of their occupational exposure to mercuric nitrate.

There are more than a hundred manufactured sources of mercury pollution in America.[78] One of the worst is the methyl mercury contamination of many freshwater and seawater fish. The larger the fish, the worse the pollution, because large fish eat smaller fish that have already built up a concentration of mercury in their bodies and hence increase their own mercury levels. Yellowfin and big-eye tuna and swordfish are especially affected. *Don't believe anyone who tells you they are safe.* Stick to skipjack and albacore.

By serendipity, the furor over toxic levels of mercury in large fish led recently to the discovery of a way to combat it. Some big marine mammals also high up the food chain were found to have inexplicably *low* levels of mercury.[79] Nice detective work showed that these animals had a high selenium intake. Now, it has been established that tiny amounts of dietary selenium will detoxify much larger amounts of mercury in the body, especially if combined with its complementary antioxidant, Vitamin E.[80]

What a superb example of the precision that nature invested in the design of humanity. If mercury builds up, the body has the precise mechanism to change the metabolism of selenium and build it up too, provided it is available in the diet. Though selenium is essential in minute amounts, in the presence of a mercury burden the body will accumulate it to toxic levels. Both minerals then remain in the body *and detoxify each other.*[81] And yet some ignoble scientists still claim that human nutrition is a simple matter!

Lead is different. Despite the uproar over car-exhaust lead filling our urban air, we get far more lead pollution from our diet.[82] The supposedly safe levels of lead in foods have been progressively lowered over the years as more and more diseases are found to be connected with lead burden, especially in children. Although its 1980 "guidelines" are still used, the FDA is no longer sure that *any* level of lead is safe.[83] For a five-year-old the *maximum* tolerable intake in the guidelines is 150 mcg per day. If you give your child a lot of canned foods, including soups, meats, fish and vegetables, you can easily exceed this figure. In 1981 *Consumer Reports* found that one 4-oz serving of canned beans contained between 50 and 60 mcg of lead.[84] It will take years yet for the FDA to push through its proposed legislation to get the lead out of cans. Meanwhile, eating most canned foods is a slow, sure form of poisoning. Progressive lead pollution leads to anemia, kidney, thyroid and heart damage, and degeneration of the brain.[85]

Nutritional deficiencies increase lead effects. Low levels of zinc, iron, calcium and phosphorus, likely in many Americans, allow lead to enter the body. The deficiencies need to be only marginal to greatly enhance lead absorption.[86] Conversely, supplementation with these minerals, especially iron and zinc, reverses lead poisoning.[87] It has just been established that Vitamin E supplements may also reduce lead poisoning.[88] But don't wait to be poisoned. The best line of defense against all unavoidable toxic substances in our environment is continuous optimum nutrition.

We cannot cover all the food additives and other environmental pollutants in this book. Nor can we cover the additive effects of many pollutants acting simultaneously against the human body. Nevertheless, even the brief examples given show that the levels of toxic pollutants in our food and environment so increase the body's needs for nutrients that the needs of an American citizen today no longer bear any relation to the standards of nutrients required in a benign environment, or nutrients required simply to prevent certain deficiency diseases. The large number of different nutrients needed to combat different pollutants, the low levels of nutrients in our foods, our poor dietary habits and the loss of bioavailability of nutrients in the average diet all combine with our knowledge of the interdependent interactions of all nutrients to indicate that nothing short of a complete vitamin and mineral supplement will suffice.

Millions of years of evolution developed the mechanisms in the human body which give it optimum health by ingesting a certain, precise mix of natural substances. Evolution had no way of knowing that twentieth-century technology would strip our food of these nutrients so that we could be sure of obtaining them only by taking supplements. Evolution had no way of knowing that the twentieth-century human body would also be deluged with toxic pollutants which increase our needs for nutrients far beyond those originally prescribed by nature. Our only defense is to use nutrition science to design vitamin and mineral supplements to suit each individual's unique biochemistry and unique life situation. It can be done, and it will be done in the twenty-first century. By *carefully* following this book, you can start to do it today.

CHAPTER 4

YOU CAN INHIBIT AGING

THE MOST WIDESPREAD degenerative disease in America today is premature old age. *It is also the most preventable.* But the knowledge required to prevent it is recent and scattered over a number of scientific fields. Like most Western countries, America has retarded applied science by rewarding the specialization of research rather than the synthesis needed to apply it.[1] It is a double-edged error. By inhibiting the application of knowledge about aging, we lose our best decision-makers to senility or death when their accumulated wisdom is at a peak no younger person can match. It's about time we used what is known to help them—and us—to live longer, healthier lives.

The idea of prolonging life evokes grisly images because geriatric medicine is concentrated on preventing death or insanity in elderly sick people. But most of us are not interested in the extra few years of lingering degeneration provided by medical life-supports. We want to extend the duration of vital health. We want to be skiing at eighty, dancing at a hundred. Extension of maximum lifespan must follow, because *it is disease that kills us, not chronological age.*

Inhibiting aging is not difficult. Like the prevention of degenerative disease, it does not require supertechnology, exotic drugs or magic potions. Nothing proposed here is very demanding, nor do you need to become a saint. Provided you are not in the grip of a degenerative disease already, you are likely to get at least an extra decade of vigorous years, and perhaps a lot more, added to your life, *no matter what age you are now.*

Lifespan Is Not Necessarily Limited

Until recently, it was widely believed that aging was a timeclock mechanism giving life a fixed limit laid down in the genes. Famous gerontologist Dr. Leonard Hayflick, now a medical professor at the University of Florida, showed that human cell cultures grown in a dish could divide a limited number of times. This *fibroblast replicative limit,* as it is called, suggested that the human cell has an inbuilt timing mechanism which limits its life.[2] But other scientists were suspicious of Hayflick's conclusion, because of widespread evidence that mutation in human cells produces cultures that have an unlimited number of divisions, that is, are potentially immortal.

My favorite is the HE-LA strain, named after its donor, *He*nrietta *La*cks, who died of cancer in 1951. Henrietta bequeathed some of her cells to science for cancer research. They are now sent all over the world for this purpose. Far from showing signs of dying, her cells grow stronger year by year. Stray HE-LA cells that happen to get on laboratory glassware invade other cell cultures, destroy them and take their place. For years cell cultures going from one laboratory to another have inadvertently distributed HE-LA cells to such an extent that they now turn up everywhere. Cultures that are supposed to be bone cells, kidney cells or stomach cells all turn out to be HE-LA. Commercial cell cultures and even individual laboratory cultures have been contaminated so badly that there is now a special project run by Dr. Walter Nelson Rees at the University of California to track down the immortal HE-LA as they thrive in laboratories from London to Los Angeles.[3]

So, we are pretty sure the timeclock theory of lifespan is wrong. More likely, the ability of cells to reproduce themselves depends on the adequacy of their nutrition. If there is the slightest inadequacy in the nutrient medium in which they are grown, then deficits will gradually accumulate to damage cells and impair their function. Hospital patients who have to be fed intravenously provide an illustration of this. Their liquid "food" is made with ample amounts of all the accepted essential nutrients. But it is not good enough. Because nutrients cannot work properly if even one is missing, these patients develop all sorts of deficiencies. Until about ten years ago, one of these was chromium deficiency. A patient would seem well nourished for months, then gradually developed deterioration of the peripheral nerves and impaired glucose tolerance. Today we know chromium is an essential element, so doctors add a few *millionths* of a gram of chromium to the nutrient formula. This corrects the deficit, and the symptoms disappear.[4] Unfortunately, we do not know the perfect artificial nutrient formula for human beings or for cell cultures, so it is likely that the replicative limit found in laboratory studies of human cells reflects this ignorance more than it demonstrates a life-timing mechanism.

The second reason to doubt the notion of inbuilt clocks comes from the ongoing research of Dr. R. Holliday and his colleagues at the British National Institute for Medical Research.[5] Cells do not all divide all the time, and many human cells may live for very long periods without division. If replicating cells have a maximum life of, say, 100 years, then identical cells in that population that do not replicate for 30 years have a potential life of 130 years. So, even if there is a replicative limit, which is doubtful, it is not the same as a lifespan limit.

The human body is not like the "Wonderful One-Hoss Shay" of Oliver Wendell Holmes. It is not fixed in structure and function. It does not age all together. Rather, the body is a dynamic expression of the life process, continually re-creating itself out of the raw materials it ingests. If we could nourish it perfectly and prevent it from being damaged, there is no evidence to contradict the idea that a human being would live indefinitely We are a long way from achieving this potential, but leading gerontologists believe that people older than the 120 legendary years of Moses will be commonplace by the twenty-first century.[6]

The graphs in Figure 2 show the likely development. The percentage of the population living at each age is indicated by the falling line. The line showing the mortality of the American population in 1900 indicates that 20 percent died at birth or in early childhood. More than half the population died before age sixty. The 1979 mortality line shows that advances of medical science in saving babies have reduced childhood deaths to a very small percentage. Improvements in nutrition, sanitation, housing and immunization, plus a contribution from antibiotics, now keep 80 percent of the population alive until age sixty. But beyond age sixty, there is a rapid mortality rate, and the maximum lifespan in 1979 is little different from that in 1900.

Until now, the effects of science have been felt by younger people (the top of the curve). The last line represents a reasonable projection of mortality in the year 2020 if the scientific advances discussed in this chapter are generally adopted. As you can see, they favor people at older ages by shifting the bottom of the curve out so that 40 percent of the population reaches 100 years, and the maximum lifespan is 125 years. Let us hope we are ready for the social consequences.

Exercise Inhibits Aging

The human body evolved to be continuously active when not sleeping. Yet modern life is so sedentary, we are in danger of losing the use of our legs. People who lead purely sedentary lives lose muscle and bone so fast that they should have frequent medical examinations to monitor the inevitable physical degeneration caused by the stress of all that inactivity.

Together with adequate nutrition, correct, regular exercise confers many benefits. It increases your metabolic rate and reduces body fat, thereby helping to prevent obesity, the harbinger of many degenerative diseases.[7] It maintains your lean mus-

Figure 2: Existing and projected mortality curves for the United States

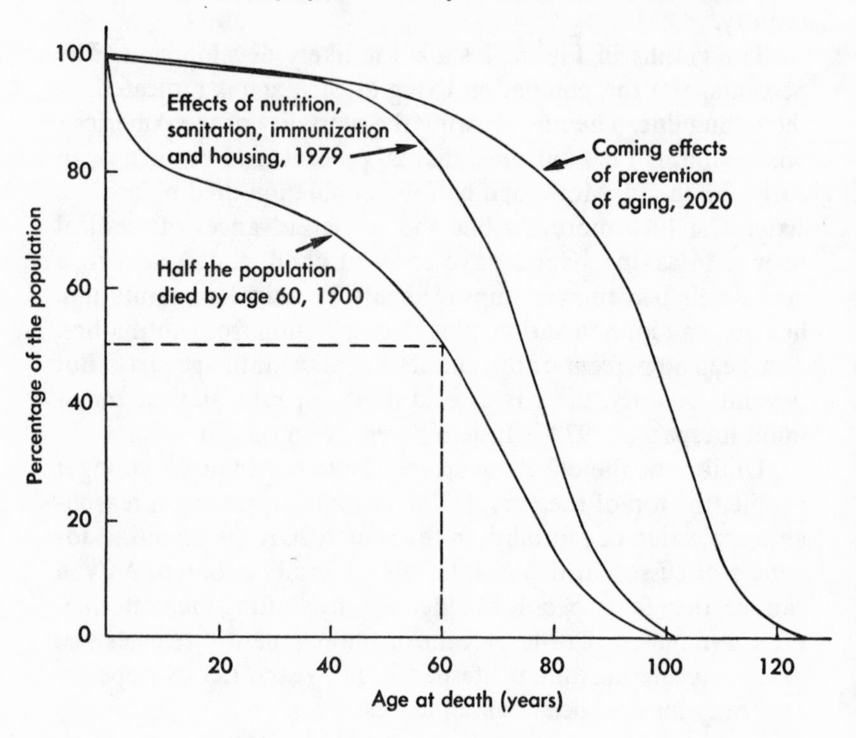

cle mass and your skeletal frame, both of which otherwise decline rapidly with aging.[8] Exercise also protects the cardiovascular system against otherwise inevitable atherosclerosis,[9] and maintains peripheral circulation and optimum oxygenation of tissue, combating the development of circulatory problems characteristic of aging.[10] It protects glucose tolerance against the degenerative changes that lead to adult-onset diabetes,[11] and prevents the rise in blood pressure which accompanies aging in America.[12] Finally, exercise maintains reaction speed and produces substances in the blood which relieve anxiety and depression.[13] It would be very surprising, then, if it didn't prolong healthy life.

Yet some well-known studies have concluded that exercise

does not extend lifespan. Fortunately, there is a great deal wrong with this research. The popular method is to examine the death records of athletes. The most comprehensive analysis was published in 1979 by Dr. Anthony Polednak.[14] In one of the studies he reviewed, 629 athletes who were varsity letter men at Michigan State University were compared with 583 nonathletes. There was no difference in longevity between the groups. A larger examination of 6,300 Harvard athletes (letter men) found that they died significantly *earlier* than nonathletes. The basic fault with these studies is that there is no evidence that the athletes continued to exercise after they left their sport, or even after they left the university. For many, their exercise habits were linked to group training with the team. When no longer on the team, they may have stopped exercising entirely.

In 1979 we questioned one hundred team athletes at the University of Auckland. Only thirty-four of them continued to work out or do any kind of training in the off-season. In fact, the majority were so unfit for half the year that we had to reject team players as possible participants in our vitamin studies. We used track and field athletes instead, individual sportsmen who train year-round. If most team athletes, who constitute the majority of the letter men in the longevity studies, do not exercise during off-seasons, they are unlikely to do so later in life. So, studies of deceased university athletes have no bearing on exercise and lifespan because there is no evidence that the ex-athletes did any.

Certainly, exercise done in the past puts a certain amount of credit in your health bank. But once you stop exercising, the body deteriorates rapidly. With only twenty-four hours of inactivity, muscle tissue starts to deteriorate.[15] That is why you are too weak to walk properly after only a few days in bed. Another good example is the wasting of muscles that occurs with lack of use after a broken arm or leg is put in a cast. With a year of inactivity, more than half the physiological benefit of an athletic career is gone. Within five years of sedentary life, ex-athletes have no physiological advantage left over people who have never exercised. In fact, they may be worse off, because of that bane of the ex-athlete—overweight. Reduced activity levels no longer match the gargantuan appetites shaped during the years of sporting glory, and the pounds roll on.

The only studies that do illustrate the effects of exercise on aging are those that measure activity throughout life. An excellent study was completed in 1977 by Drs. Charles Rose and Michel Cohen of the Veterans Administration Hospital in Boston, Massachusetts.[16] They traced the death records of five hundred white males who had died in Boston, and who had living relatives who could give information on their exercise habits during life. Seventy percent of the informants were wives and 20 percent were children of the deceased, so there was a reasonable chance of obtaining accurate information. Their exercise level, both on the job and during leisure hours, was rated on a scale ranging from sedentary to very active. Job exercise was included because it is commonly thought that some jobs are strenuous enough to provide sufficient exercise. Both types of exercise fell rapidly with age, with leisure time exercise declining to "light" (one step above "sedentary") by age sixty-nine. On-the-job exercise was fairly constant up to age forty, then declined rapidly. Job exercise was not correlated with longevity at all, giving the lie to the old myth. In contrast, those who continued a high level of leisure-time exercise lived 7.1 years longer than those whose leisure exercise declined from a high level in their twenties to a low level by their forties. *Continued* exercise throughout life extends lifespan.

Further support for this conclusion stems from a study of elderly athletes. The recent popularity of Masters' track-and-field athletics contests has brought many oldsters into athletic training. Drs. Terence Kavanagh and Roy Shephard studied 128 men and 7 women who participated in the 1975 World Masters' Championships in Toronto.[17] Many were not champion athletes but simply average individuals who continued to exercise even at an advanced age (up to ninety years old). These people showed much less evidence of aging than the average person.

After age thirty, people generally lose height by about half an inch per decade as the skeleton degenerates. The study found that the old athletes had lost less than half the usual amount, indicating considerable skeletal maintenance. Also, from the ages of forty to ninety, they had less body fat, better musculature and better lung and heart function than people of the same ages in the general population. None of the participants in the Masters' Championships were using individually designed supplements, although some were using vitamins. That they were able to maintain their bodies under such haphazard nutrition demonstrates the strong anti-aging effects of continued exercise.

You don't have to be an athlete to benefit from exercise. In 1969 the London Sports Council mounted a ten-year study on aging men and women who were put on a regime of moderate daily exercise.[18] Measurements in 1979 showed that the people who continued to exercise throughout had entirely prevented the usual age-related degeneration of their bone structure, muscles and cardiovascular system. By the end of the study some were over eighty!

The effects of exercise are a good illustration of the final point that must be understood in order to prevent degenerative disease and extend your lifespan—*the principle of physiological dynamics.* Your body is not a fixed structure. It changes slowly but very surely to match exactly the nutrition you give it and the exercise you give it. The nutrients you put in are half the story. The use you make of your body is the other half. You can nurture a muscle and make it function optimally. But unless you exercise it, it can function only to its present structural limits.

If you want to strengthen the muscle further you must put it under *long-term progressive overload,* so that the new cells being formed every day to replace worn-out cells conform to increased demands placed on the muscle. For example, say you use a ten-pound weight in an exercise until you can handle it easily. To strengthen the muscle further, you must then use an eleven-pound weight, then twelve pounds, and so on. The same goes for endurance. First you jog half a mile, then three quarters of a mile, then a mile. Using this system, anyone in normal health can easily gain enough endurance capacity to run a marathon.

Exercise progress is slow but sure. The body has to wait for the death of worn-out cells before it can replace them with the improved cells built in response to the exercise. Most exercise programs fail either because they are too short, or because they are not progressive. Without progressive overload you cannot continue to improve. That is why people who do the same three-mile jog and ten minutes of calisthenics five days a week for years do not get progressively fitter and stronger. It's better than doing nothing, of course, but not good enough if you want the optimum physiological benefit.

The human body is superbly adaptive. Far from becoming weaker and slower with age, it becomes weaker and slower with malnutrition, poisoning and lack of progressive exercise. There is no physiological reason that you cannot continue to improve in strength and endurance from your twenties on into your eighties. We have more to say about how to do it in Chapter 5. If you adopt a correct exercise program as part of your individual biochemical equation, you will not only ward off degenerative disease better than with nutrition alone, but you will also substantially extend your lifespan.

The Mechanisms of Aging

If we escape fatal injuries or infections, we die from the progressive accumulation of small biochemical imbalances in the body resulting from poor nutrition, accidents, illnesses and the invasion of toxic substances. Eventually, the body is sufficiently weakened so that one or another degenerative disease, silently lurking within, can take over. For the unlucky, lingering illness follows, until one or more organ systems fail. For the lucky, an organ system fails immediately. *We do not die of old age, we die of disease.*

The way to a longer, more vigorous life does not lie in medical treatment *after* disease has struck, but in prevention. Rather than resorting to drugs or surgery in a vain attempt to fight nature by patching a failing system, we should seek the answer given us by heredity, the answer that interlocks us with nature. That answer lies in three superb systems developed by evolution: the overall DNA code, the histocompatibility complex and the immune system. These sytems renew your body substance every day so it is identical to the way it was yesterday, prevent invasion of the body by degenerative disease, repair the body after injury and eject foreign toxins.

Your body has a unique identity code, the histocompatibility complex, whose sole function is to protect you. It enables the body to mobilize the immune system to attack and destroy any invader. When it is working well, neither disease nor poison can remain active in the body. In concert with the histocompatibility complex, you have a DNA coding system contained in the nucleus of each of the *sixty trillion* cells that make up your body. This coding system tells the body exactly what to make to renew cells and intercellular substances as they wear out.

Every day, for example, your body makes about one million red blood cells to replace those that wear out and die. Because of your DNA code, it makes them identical to previous cells. The same goes for hair and hands, eyes and toes. Each year, most of the cells in your body are renewed. The DNA system ensures they are renewed exactly as before. Think of it this way. Each year, you grow a new nose; the DNA code keeps it exactly the same shape as the old one. Only when damage to the DNA disrupts its functions do the characteristic changes of age begin to appear.

The conquest of aging involves the preventive maintenance of the DNA code, and of the histocompatibility complex and its troops, the immune system. If you begin the conquest after age twenty, it also means repairing any damage that has already occurred to these systems. In the last five years medical science has discovered some of the mechanisms involved in these repairs. As might be expected of nature, they are all interrelated.

DNA damage accumulates with aging.[19] If DNA damage is deliberately induced, aging is accelerated. In 1974 Drs. Ronald Hart and Richard Setlow showed that longevity is correlated with the capacity to repair DNA damage in species ranging from mouse to man. Humans are the longest-lived primates and have the best DNA repair capacity.[20] In a breakthrough reported in 1979, Dr. Joan Smith-Sonneborn of the University of Wyoming used certain wavelengths and exposures of light to boost DNA repair in a single-celled creature called Paramecium. The DNA was repaired so well that the Paramecium lifespan *was extended by 50 percent.*[21] This was the first demonstration that science can directly intervene to rejuvenate a normal organism and extend its lifespan.

The use of light to reactivate repair enzymes also works to rejuvenate human skin. Your skin is as sensitive to light as the petals of a flower. But it is a huge leap from rejuvenation of skin cells to rejuvenation of a human being. Just lying under the ultraviolet, be it the sun or the ray-lamp, *accelerates* human aging. Nevertheless, there is other compelling evidence that DNA repair promotes longevity and that this repair capacity is linked to the histocompatibility complex. In 1977 Dr. Roy Walford and his colleagues at UCLA Medical School studied fourteen different strains of mice that were genetically identical except for differences in their histocompatibility complex. The lifespan of the mice varied directly with these differences.[22] The mice with the greatest DNA repair capacity also lived the longest.[23] So the histocompatibility complex is connected with DNA repair capacity, which in turn is a major determinant of lifespan.

The repair capacity of DNA is also linked to the strength of the immune system. The shortest-lived strain of mice, the NZB mouse, is the classic model used in laboratory research for the study of immunological defects. The NZB mouse has an immune system that is weak and easily damaged. In contrast, the longest-lived strain, the CBA mouse, has the strongest immune system.[24]

Given these links between the three systems and longevity,

we can build a picture of how aging probably works. Shortly after puberty in a "healthy" person, damage to DNA (and its associated RNA systems) starts to accumulate. The DNA code begins to produce slightly altered cells, especially in damaged areas of the body, and characteristic age changes appear. The histocompatibility complex may fail to recognize the altered cells and if so, will order an immune-system attack on them, causing further damage.

The histocompatibility complex itself accumulates damage, and its identity code becomes less precise. So it starts failing to recognize foreign invading cells and toxins, and fails to instruct the immune system to destroy them. Eventually, the histocompatibility complex code is so damaged that the immune system starts producing *autoantibodies,* rogue troops that will attack normal cells. The slight alterations in normal cells resulting from DNA damage makes them harder to recognize, thereby also enhancing the probability of the body attacking itself. The number of autoantibodies increases rapidly with age,[25] bringing with them the continual threat of cancer, which is simply cells that do not recognize their place in the body's scheme. The concentration of these cells in the body is highly correlated with smoking, with degenerative diseases, especially cardiovascular disease, and with premature death.[26]

Meanwhile, the immune system itself accumulates damage. It becomes less able to carry out the search-and-destroy instructions of the histocompatibility complex, and foreign cells and substances start to accumulate. As the strength of the immune system declines, so vulnerability to degenerative disease increases.[27] By seventy years of age, your immune system may have lost 90 percent of its fighting capacity.

Preventing the Damage of Aging

To inhibit aging, we have to prevent the interrelated damage to these vital systems. We don't know everything yet, but we know enough to make a good start. In humans, chromosome Number 6 in the genes contains the histocompatibility complex. It also contains the regulators for our enzyme systems, the biological catalysts that destroy toxins and maintain our cellular identity.[28] One of these regulators linked to the histocompatibility complex controls the production of important protective enzymes called superoxide dismutases (SODs). SODs protect us against the toxic effects of oxygen. Yes, oxygen. Although it is vital to life, oxygen is also poisonous. The use of oxygen creates toxic by-products, highly reactive substances called *superoxides* or *free radicals,* which can damage any part of the body, including the immune system itself, the histocompatibility complex and even the DNA code secreted in the cell nucleus. SODs destroy superoxides. Dr. Richard Cutler of the National Institute on Aging has shown that the SOD level in primates is highly correlated with longevity.[29] Laboratories are now supplementing animal diets with SODs in an attempt to increase lifespan. As yet there is *no* reliable evidence that dietary SOD will increase its levels in the blood or that it prolongs life.[30]

SOD in the diet would have a hard time getting into the body, because it is such a large molecule that it can hardly fit through the holes in cell membranes. So, assuming that dietary SOD survives the digestive process intact, and then somehow gets through the intestine walls, its action in the body is confined to boosting SOD activity in the spaces between cells. This may have an effect in protecting the cell membranes themselves from external free-radical damage by surrounding them with SOD troops that destroy free radicals on contact. If so, it could be important, because cell membranes deteriorate with age, and their structural integrity is *the* best protective device against cell damage. We await the evidence. Until there is some, the over-the-counter SODs being widely promoted by pharmacies and health-food stores are just commercial gobbledegook.

A prescription preparation of SOD that can be injected into the bloodstream is being used in the experimental drug treatment of cancer, arthritis, radiation poisoning and muscular dystrophy under the generic name "Orgotein," or the trade name "Ontosein." It is of possible value in such a wide variety of degenerative diseases because damaging superoxides in the body aggravate the inflammatory reactions present in many diseases. SODs destroy superoxides or render them inactive and thereby reduce inflammation. The injectable form may work because at least it gets into the bloodstream intact.

The biggest value of discovery of the SOD mechanism is the clues it gives us about the damaging effects of oxygen on the human body. Some two billion years ago, when plant life started to cover the earth and release a lot of free oxygen, this excess of oxygen killed all organisms except those that developed mechanisms to deal with oxygen poisoning. We still have those ancient SOD mechanisms in all our cells. Their link with the histocompatibility complex, the body's master defense control, indicates their importance in maintaining the body. It also underscores the importance of preventing free-radical accumulation in the system, whether it be from our use of oxygen or from other sources, such as the oxidation of fats or the ultraviolet radiation in sunlight.

Fortunately, we do not have to rely on SOD. During evolution the body also developed mechanisms to use the nutrient antioxidants, Vitamins C and E and selenium, as free-radical controllers. They are very effective against all sources of free radicals.[31] Radiation, for example, damages the body by creating masses of free radicals. Dietary C and E and especially selenium offer protection against levels of radiation that otherwise would kill you within seventy-two hours.[32] With the rumble of Three Mile Island still shaking our bones, nutrient antioxidants are sensible precautions for the radiation reason alone.

The studies using these antioxidants to increase lifespan have had mixed results. In mice, antioxidants in the diet have resulted only in fewer deposits of the brown fatty age pigment (lipofuscin) that is a characteristic sign on the skin of all aging mammals.[33] These "age spots" also form inside the body and interfere with all its functions. There is some evidence that the mice who consumed antioxidants were also more vigorous and less diseased in old age than those whose diet did not include antioxidants. But they didn't live much longer.

The only other reasonable study of the effects of antioxidants on lifespan was done on cells grown in laboratory cultures. In 1975 Drs. Lester Packer and James Smith at the University of California caused a lot of excitement by *doubling* the lifespan of cells by adding Vitamin E to the nutrient medium in which the cells were grown.[34] This finding, often called a breakthrough by vitamin faddists, is cited as evidence that Vitamin E retards aging. What the enthusiasts don't mention is that neither Packer and Smith nor anyone else has been able to repeat these results.[35] Vitamin E alone does not extend lifespan.

Why did these studies fail? Probably because no one used a complete nutrient supplement. They expected antioxidants to work on their own without the complementary nutrients evolution made essential to their function. Our laboratory at the University of Auckland has done a preliminary study suggesting that the lifelong addition of complete supplements to the diet extends the lifespan of laboratory rats by up to 30 percent. A comprehensive study to confirm this finding is now under way. There is a high probability of success, because a complete supplement of vitamins and minerals inhibits aging not only by preventing free-radical damage, but also in many other ways. One of these is through the nutrients' effects in maintaining the immune system.

Most degenerative diseases are accompanied by damage to the immune system. A defective immune system is implicated in all diseases that produce premature aging, such as systemic lupus, which afflicts half a million Americans, and Alzheimer's disease (premature senility).[36] In most of these cases the immune system gradually becomes defective over many years. We know the immune system is connected with premature aging because of studies done on strains of animals born with a defective immune system. The NZB strain of mouse is one example. This wee fellow has only a third the lifespan of other similar mice, and is terribly subject to all the "aging" diseases.

NZB mice give us valuable clues about aging. They have a specific defect in the white-cell system of body defenders, a defect in what are called T-lymphocytes or T-cells. These are our main mechanism of cellular immunity. Keeping the T-cells in top condition is critical to the prevention of aging. They protect the body against foreign cells, bacteria, fungi, viruses and allergens. They also help the body resist cancer and the autoimmune diseases we discussed earlier. Defective T-cell function accompanies most degenerative diseases, including cancers, rheumatoid arthritis, multiple sclerosis, diabetes mellitus and ulcerative colitis. A big part of aging is the gradual decline in T-cells, which occurs even without any apparent disease.[37] So if vitamins and minerals can maintain this essential part of the immune system, we are well on the way to inhibiting aging.

Vitamin C Protects the Immune System

T-cells have a very high level of Vitamin C. With age degeneration, the level drops progressively,[38] and we lose our resistance to disease. The Vitamin C level of T-cells (and companion white cells) is essential in fighting disease, because if you do get a virus or other infection, it drops very quickly.[39] After you recover, T-cells slowly build up their Vitamin C again.[40] The more severe the infection, the worse the loss, unless you take a C supplement. Dietary Vitamin C reduces the loss of T-cell C and can considerably reduce symptoms.[41]

Smoking, which puts the body under severe stress, provides further evidence that Vitamin C supplements are needed to maintain T-cells. The Vitamin C level of T-cells (and of companion white cells) is very low in smokers, and so is their resistance to disease. Dietary supplements of C restore the level to normal.[42]

It may take many thousand milligrams of Vitamin C to restore T-cells to normal, especially in someone who has a virus.[43] And the action of T-cells continues to improve as you increase the amount of C.[44] This recent knowledge goes a long way toward explaining the controversy over Vitamin C and the common cold. Over seventy studies have been done to test Dr. Linus Pauling's original theory that Vitamin C supplements prevent colds. Each year, we review them, and each year we are amazed that some physicians still do not accept the positive evidence. All the studies that have turned out negative have used inadequate amounts of Vitamin C. All have used less than 4,000 mg a day. When we know that infection severely depletes reserves of C, and that some people without colds may need more than 5,000 mg a day just for normal functioning, then the failure of studies using smaller amounts is very likely.

Another major fault of the negative studies is their unnatural methods of infection. In three studies that are much quoted against the Pauling theory, infection was carried out by squirting virulent laboratory-bred cold viruses up the noses of the hapless subjects. Then they were given three grams of Vitamin C a day.[45] That is like testing a boxer's mouth guard by hitting him in the teeth with a sledgehammer. Three grams of C is woefully insufficient against a viral attack so huge that it would never occur in normal life. There is no longer any doubt of the benefit of C supplements against the common cold,[46] even though the Vitamin C has to rely on the diet for its complementary nutrients.

In normal healthy mice and healthy human subjects, large supplements of Vitamin C improve the action of T-cells in protecting the body.[47] This is especially interesting in mice because, unlike human beings, they produce their own Vitamin C. Even so, supplementary C can improve mouse resistance to disease. Collaborative studies are just being designed in my laboratory on animals, and in Walter Reed Hospital in Washington on patients undergoing surgery, to determine whether supplementary

Vitamin C given *before* the body is put under stress will protect the immune system.

From even the few studies reviewed, it seems clear that ample Vitamin C is required to maintain the T-cells and our resistance to disease. From Chapter 3 we know that some individuals may need more than 5,000 mg of C a day. Yet there is no way to obtain even 1,000 mg from any normal diet today. So in order to maintain the optimum immune function essential to the inhibition of aging, it is necessary for each one of us to use extra C and its complementary nutrients every day.

The B Vitamins Protect the Immune System

In the laboratory, animals are "challenged" with various diseases to examine the effects of vitamins on their immune systems. Deficiencies of Vitamins B_1 (thiamine), B_2 (riboflavin), B_3 (niacin) and the cofactor (helper substance) biotin reduce resistance markedly. If B_5 (pantothenic acid) or B_6 (pyridoxine) are deficient, resistance drops almost to zero.[48] As we have seen, these two B vitamins are widely deficient in the American diet. So the common practice of taking Vitamin C alone to ward off infections just cannot work properly. Without the complementary nutrients B_1, B_2, B_3, B_5 and B_6 (and others we haven't discussed), the immune system cannot do its job.

Some people tell me, "Oh, I take a B complex as well," or "I take a multivitamin too." Unfortunately, 99 percent of these people have no idea what B vitamins are included in the supplements they take, in what amounts, in what forms, or how much is bioavailable. Even the rare woman (it's almost always a woman) who does know exactly what she is taking has no idea of how much of each B vitamin is necessary to balance the C supplement, or how much of *any* vitamin is necessary for her unique biochemical makeup.

Other B vitamins we found to be widely deficient in the

American diet are folic acid and Vitamin B_{12} (cobalamin). Folic-acid anemia is commonplace in women, and B_{12} shots now seem to be challenging martinis as the national pick-me-up. Both vitamins are involved in the maintenance of the immune system and hence in the inhibition of aging. As you might expect, their action is interrelated.[49]

In animals the white cells of the immune system we discussed in relation to Vitamin C are reduced by up to *80 percent* by folic-acid deficiency.[50] In one study, animals that were deprived of folic acid were infected with dysentery (*Shigella flexneria*), the common cause of diarrhea in humans. Nine out of every ten animals died, half of them within twenty-four hours. The control group of animals that was given ample folic acid was also given the infection. *None died.*[51] How precise is nature, when the deficiency of a few millionths of a gram of *one* micronutrient can kill. When you hear "experts" claiming vitamin supplements are unnecessary, it should remind you of overweening vanity and the Tower of Babel.

Vitamin B_{12} is also needed for folic acid to do its job. It carries folic acid into the white cells of the immune system.[52] If this transport system fails, the immune system quickly degenerates and vulnerability to disease increases and aging is accelerated. Many Americans cannot get sufficient B_{12} from their diet. Though there is probably enough B_{12} in their food, many people can't absorb even the few micrograms required each day. The absorption of B_{12} depends on a constituent of gastric juices called the "intrinsic factor." The very anemia produced by B_{12} deficiency interferes with this factor and prevents absorption. So, low B_{12} is a vicious cycle. The less the body contains, the less it can absorb. Shots of B_{12} temporarily improve matters, but as with any nutrient introduced by an unnatural route, they interfere with the body's ability to extract and process nutrients from what it eats. Far better that the body get its B_{12} through the intestine, as nature designed it to do.

One way to facilitate absorption of B_{12} is to reduce all fats in your diet. High-fat diets prevent the body from producing the intrinsic factor necessary for B_{12} absorption. This defect not only affects the immune system by supplying insufficient B_{12} for transport of folic acid, but can also lead to pernicious anemia, a life-threatening illness. These are strong reasons for reducing all fats in your diet if you want to avoid degenerative disease.

Vitamin E Protects the Immune System

Large amounts of Vitamin E also enhance our immune responses and improve resistance to disease.[53] It is heartening to see this new work showing that scientists are now recognizing the potential of Vitamin E, even though its exact functions in the body remain unknown.

Let us take just one example of Vitamin E's effects on immune function. Mice, those ever-present laboratory sacrifices to medicine, were given extra Vitamin E, then deliberately infected with pneumonia. Over 60 percent of them showed strong resistance to the disease. A control group, given only a normal mouse diet, all developed the pneumonia.[54] The important point of this study is that the normal diet, which *failed* to protect the mice, contained what was thought to be an adequate amount of Vitamin E. It took supplementation with *extra* E to protect normal, healthy animals. In 1981 world expert on Vitamin E Dr. Robert Tengerdy and his colleagues at Colorado State University concluded that proper immune function may require six times the Vitamin E previously thought to be nutritionally adequate.[55]

We have discussed only a few of the recent studies that show how important vitamin supplements are for preventive maintenance of the immune system to defend us against aging and disease. We have not touched on the effect of essential minerals, although there is increasing evidence that these too are involved. Zinc, for example, widely deficient in the American diet,[56] is essential for the maintenance of T-cells.[57] Nevertheless, even what we have covered is sufficient to indicate that you will not maintain your immune system or retard aging without a complete vitamin and mineral supplement. In the animal and human studies described, no attempt was made to use complete supplements or to design the supplement to suit the individual. If you do both, you can confidently expect even better results.

The older you start, the more carefully your supplement should be designed. Begun in middle life, nutrient supplementation has much more to do than strengthen immune function. It must also reverse the accumulation of damaging free radicals we discussed. And it must reverse any damage already done by free radicals, especially to the immune system itself and to the cardiovascular system. Past the age of forty, you probably have also accumulated some of the common defects of aging. These have to be corrected too. Nevertheless, provided you are not ill now, nutritional science can do a lot to repair you.

Undereating Retards Aging

If you are short to medium height and more than twenty pounds overweight, or medium height to tall and more than forty pounds overweight, read Chapter 8 before this section. Here, we are concerned with the strange effects of restricting calories in people of normal weight while retaining good nutrition.

Forty-odd years ago Dr. Clive McCay at Cornell University extended the lives of rats by more than 50 percent by lifelong *severe* restriction of the calories in their diets.[58] Since then, his findings have been repeated numerous times. Dr. Maurice Ross has doubled rat lifespan with the same simple technique,[59] equivalent to extending human lifespan to two hundred years. As we would expect from our previous discussion, degenerative diseases are also inhibited in these animals.

Human beings would not stand for such a regimen. Fortunately, caloric restriction need not be so severe to obtain almost the same effects. Dr. Benjamin Berg of Columbia University has reduced degenerative disease and extended the lives of rats with a lifelong restriction of calories by one third.[60] Restricted animals are also more vigorous throughout life than animals given free access to food. Remember, these studies involved restriction of calories only. Vitamins and minerals were kept ample.

All the early studies were lifelong after weaning. Early attempts to extend lifespan by starting the same restriction in adulthood were a failure. Until recently, it was thought that the diets worked by retarding maturation, giving the rat a longer childhood. Dr. Ross had shown, however, that a special restricted diet composed of one part protein to five parts calories increases lifespan in adult rats that were fed freely before adulthood.[61] The best protein-to-calorie ratio to use *for adult rats* seems to be between 1:5 and 1:8.[62] There is also evidence that gradual rather than sudden imposition of calorie restriction brings the best results in maintaining, and even rejuvenating, the immune system in adult animals.[63]

At first blush all these studies seemed to suffer a serious defect which makes the findings inapplicable to human beings. Animals used as controls lived in cages surrounded by ample food, with nothing to do but eat and sleep. These rats were plump and slow. They are quite different from the fast, lean (and often mean) rats on low-calorie diets, who look more like wild rats. It may be that the lean rats were getting the *correct amount* of food to live their normal span, and the fat rats were overeating themselves to an early death.

At second blush, however, that is what humans often do—sit around and eat. More than fifty million Americans are badly overweight. Given plenty of food, both rats and men dig their graves with their teeth. If we live longer, healthier lives by cutting down on calories, it may be because the restriction is more like the conditions under which the human body evolved. It is very likely that *Homo sapiens,* the nervous hunter of empty lands, developed a body that just cannot remain healthy if it is enveloped in blubber.

No one has been able to study adult human beings long enough yet to see for sure if caloric restriction extends our lifespan. It is a pretty safe bet though, especially as the life-extension effects in animals are accompanied by resistance to degenerative disease and rejuvenation of the immune system. The good news is that you may not have to make any real effort to reduce your caloric intake.

In 1972, at the University of Auckland and in my private clinic, we began giving overweight people individually designed vitamin and mineral supplements. Our reducing system was very successful. By 1974 we had many case reports that people felt less hungry on the regime and gradually lost weight without effort. It seemed logical, because their bodies were better nourished than before, but we were puzzled because the usual response to a reducing diet is to feel ravenous. So we compared six male long-distance runners who were very lean with six overweight people.

All twelve persons restricted their consumption of processed carbohydrates and processed fats so that their calorie intake was reduced by approximately one third. All were given individually designed vitamin and mineral supplements from two weeks before the study began. For the four weeks of the study, the athletes, usually voracious eaters, had no difficulty in eating less. All lost weight (three to five pounds) but reported that their training was unaffected. They did not feel hungry or weak from the diet. All the fatties lost weight too. But the important point is that even the lean athletes were probably eating too much on their normal diets. Improving their nutrition with extra vitamins and minerals enabled them to cut down drastically without detrimental effects.

In American society, where poor nutrition is common, many people become overweight because they are undernourished. Their bodies use all the powerful internal mechanisms to signal, "Keep eating, keep eating," in an attempt to get the missing nutrients. The usual response is to eat more and more processed food, which further robs the body of nutrients, thereby *increasing* the body's cry for more food. So the vicious cycle continues and fat accumulates.

We have been recording the phenomenon of individual supplements reducing the appetite of people on reducing diets for eight years. It is certainly reliable. So if you want to underfeed a bit to inhibit aging, then slowly reduce the calories by eliminating processed foods little by little over a period of a year. If you find yourself hungry or weak, you are cutting down too quickly. Provided your diet (plus supplements) is nutritionally adequate, you will not have to make yourself a martyr. Optimum nutrition should reduce your appetite (and your weight) automatically.

Maintaining the Mind

Mental degeneration is a biochemical disturbance just like physical degeneration. Eating a few millionths of a gram of LSD will demonstrate this fact to anyone. Within an hour every cell of the brain is disordered, producing the hallucinations, paranoia and other characteristics of a schizophrenic reaction. Fortunately, this chemical psychosis is usually reversible. Not so easily reversible is the mental illness produced by long-term malnutrition or by poisoning the brain with the toxic metals or other toxic substances in our food.

Unfortunately, many people still labor under the shibboleths of Freudian dogmatism that what goes on in the mind is somehow separate from the functions of the brain. Freud himself acknowledged many times that his emphasis on the mental rather than the physical causes of madness was purely a temporary measure, until science found out enough about the physical mechanisms.[64] Today we know a considerable amount about these mechanisms. For the last twenty years science has been minutely documenting relationships between the physical state of the brain and mental degeneration, and how to prevent it with optimum nutrition.[65] Unfortunately, it will take at least another twenty years for this knowledge to become the basis of practice in mental hospitals. Meanwhile, you can easily apply it yourself.

In 1980 the National Institute on Aging issued a statement in the *Journal of the American Medical Association* entitled "Senility Reconsidered." The purpose was to call to the attention of health professionals how the brain may slowly develop impairment of intellectual functions (dementia) or abruptly show significant changes in mental state (delirium). The article pointed out that many curable physical disorders produce intellectual impairment that is difficult to distinguish from irreversible brain degeneration.[66]

A little later, in September 1980, Dr. Richard Hall and his colleagues at the University of Texas Medical School published an account of one hundred mental patients who were given special, intensive physical examinations. Almost half the patients were found to have *physical* illnesses that directly caused or greatly increased their mental symptoms, and that were responsible for their admission to a mental hospital. Of these patients, 61 percent showed rapid disappearance of mental symptoms when their underlying physical disorder was treated.[67] Nutritional problems, including folic-acid deficiency, overactive thyroid, severe anemia, hypoglycemia, dehydration, iron-deficiency anemia and general malnutrition, were found to be involved in many of these cases. Bodily pollution, including prescribed drug side effects and toxic mineral poisoning, was also involved in a number of cases. And these patients were tested only for a few of the possible vitamin and mineral deficiencies and toxic-substance poisonings.

The system for calculating your nutrient supplement needs described in Chapter 6 takes account of forty-eight different nutritional variables related to mental health. With such a wide variety of nutritional deficits and poisons that can cause mental illness, we will be able to cover only brief examples of them here. A very important factor is the unnecessary use of prescribed drugs. Each year, over one million Americans are admitted to the hospital because of the side effects of prescribed drugs.[68] In 1979 the Surgeon General reported that numerous cases of apparent senility are caused by prescribed drugs and the interactions of different prescribed drugs.[69] As he points out, "Older people frequently receive too much medication. Often fewer kinds of medications and lower dosages will suffice."[70]

Prescribed drugs can cause anything from mild depression and anxiety to full-blown psychosis.[71] One of the worst consequences is that other people, including physicians, may believe you have gone insane and are no longer capable of rational judgments about your own health. As a primary preventive measure in maintaining the mind, if you are taking *any* long-term medication, request at regular intervals that your physician review its necessity and dosage.

Failing memory is a frequent symptom of brain degeneration that originates from drug or toxic-metal poisoning or nutritional deficit. One potent cause relates to a decline in the effectiveness or quantity of the brain transmitter-chemical acetylcholine, which transmits nerve impulses from one neuron to another.[72] Acetylcholine is formed from choline in the diet and acetic acid in the body. At first it seemed too easy a solution to simply increase choline in the diet to increase acetylcholine in the brain. But surprisingly, it works. The best dietary source of choline is lecithin. Rats fed lecithin granules show large, rapid increases in brain acetylcholine.[73] Sometimes nature allows us an easy win.

Unfortunately, increased acetylcholine does not necessarily mean restored memory. Tests have been done with patients who have Alzheimer's senility, a major symptom of which is profound loss of memory. Dr. W. D. Boyd and his colleagues gave patients with Alzheimer's five grams of choline chloride for two weeks. There were no improvements in memory.[74] Dr. S. H. Ferris gave other patients with moderate memory degeneration up to twenty grams of choline chloride a day for four weeks. They showed no improvements either.[75] Other studies have found positive results. In 1979 Dr. Richard Mohs and his colleagues did a study at the Palo Alto VA Hospital in California with elderly healthy people who had mild memory degeneration. With sixteen grams of choline chloride for seven days, *some* showed memory improvement.[76]

There are two problems with these studies which you should be familiar with by now. First, none used a complete nutrient supplement. They expected choline, a simple dietary cofactor of the B vitamins, to work on its own to correct a complex disturbance of brain function that undoubtedly involves multiple nutrients. Second, the researchers did not know which or how many of the patients had suffered brain damage. It is usless to increase a brain neurotransmitter if clumps of the nerve cells across which it would transmit are dead. Brain cells rarely regenerate, and certainly not in the brief periods of these studies.

Evidence that irreversible brain damage is probably a critical factor in preventing recovery from memory loss comes from a recent study in Paris at the Hôpital de la Salpêtrière. Dr. J. L. Signoret and his colleagues gave three groups of patients with Alzheimer's disease nine grams of choline citrate daily. Patients who had had the disease four years or more, and who were therefore likely to be brain damaged, showed little improvement. Patients aged fifty-nine to sixty-four years who were in the early stages of Alzheimer's improved their memories considerably.[77] This evidence provides a good illustration of a general principle for maintaining the mind: Begin early, before brain damage makes medical treatment inevitable, and probably unsuccessful.

We will look at one final example of the delicate balance between the mind and nutrition, the important new knowledge that what you are thinking influences your resistance to disease. For years "hard-nosed" scientists like myself have looked indulgently at "soft" reports that "serene mental attitude" or "cheerfulness," or similar imprecise factors, can inhibit aging and disease. Now, we have to admit that hard evidence is surfacing to support these psychological notions. One important study was completed recently by Dr. R. W. Bartrop and his colleagues at the University of New South Wales and St. Vincent's

Hospital in Sydney, Australia.[78] They examined the immune function of both men and women for six weeks after the death of their spouses. Even though some of these deaths were not sudden and unexpected but were from long-term chronic diseases, all the bereaved showed continued depression of T-cell function throughout the study. As we discussed previously, T-cells constitute our major immune-system mechanism for resistance to disease. The grief of bereavement, an emotion generated solely in the mind, was making these people vulnerable to disease and degeneration. Clearly, this purely mental stress had increased their needs for the specific nutrients that maintain immune function. Such physical consequences of grief may be responsible for the frequent death of one spouse within a few weeks of the other in older people. On the positive side, the cheerfulness and optimistic outlook characteristic of people who live to a great age may be essential to maintaining their bodies.

There Is No Programmed Death

Your lifespan is in your own hands. The rate of aging is proportional to the deficits you permit to build up. To inhibit aging, you must preserve the DNA code, the histocompatibility complex and the immune system. To accomplish this task requires optimum nutrition and the avoidance of bodily pollution. If you are past twenty years of age, you need additional nutritional supplements because of damage that has already occurred. Take heart, the evidence is good that much of this damage can be reversed.

To preserve the structure of the body also requires continued exercise throughout life. This idea of daily exercise is abhorrent to many adults. They feel that way primarily because their bodies are too defective to exercise without severe discomfort. But you don't have to huff and puff at a health club. Start very lightly and follow the system given in Chapter 5. Your body will respond magnificently.

Colleagues reading this chapter have asked me how I can ignore the thousands of papers documenting degeneration in humans through aging alone, degeneration that appears to be independent of deficit or disease. They seem to forget that *the passgage of time is a measure, not a force.* Age changes are determined by comparing average individuals of different ages. But average people are functioning far below the optimum because of their malnutrition and their bodily pollution. These defects, not time, are the forces of degeneration. So the measures are incorrect. Only now is science defining the conditions necessary for optimum human lifespan. The textbooks will have to be rewritten. After forty years of research on longevity, world-famous gerontologist Dr. Johan Bjorksten concluded in July 1981, "There is no programmed death."[79]

CHAPTER 5

SUPERIOR PHYSICAL AND MENTAL PERFORMANCE

DON'T JUMP INTO A vigorous exercise program which involves health clubs and special periods out of your working day. It has a 95 percent probability of failure. It takes too much of your time. It becomes an added burden. To get a half-hour of aerobic dance may cost another one and a half hours of traveling, changing and showering time, adding a ten-hour burden of "overtime" every week. And it's no good loading all your exercise into one day a week. It doesn't work. To be successful, exercise must be incorporated into your normal routine. Ten minutes a day when you rise in the mornings is far better physiologically than five hours at a gym on Saturdays.

Start easy. You don't need complicated machines or super-gadgets. You can exercise anywhere. Your own body weight and gravity provide ample resistance. Gradual, progressive exercise is best. There is no need to strain, no need to work to your limit. A world-famous physiologist at UCLA, Dr. Laurence Moorehouse, found that even among athletes, the strainers were self-defeating.[1] We find the same. Often they spend more time in injury than in training. You are limited by the rhythms of nature. Adaptation is slow—but sweetly sure. The first day you begin exercising, even after doing none for thirty years, your body starts to rejuvenate.

Exercise has three basic aims. First, to improve your flexibility. Degeneration means getting stiffer. Stiffness means vulnerability to all sorts of strains, sprains and skeletal disorders. Second, to improve your muscular strength and endurance. The maintenance of the muscular system is essential for extending healthy life. Third, to improve your cardiovascular condition. Good nutrition is of little use if you allow your heart and blood vessels to degenerate.

There are many good exercise books giving excellent routines for flexibility and strength. Unless you are an athlete striving for top performance, ten minutes' exercise a day is sufficient to prevent degeneration. For strength, slowly increase the *amount* of resistance week by week. For endurance, slowly increase the *duration* of resistance. For flexibility move joints *gently* to their limits and hold the pose fifteen seconds. Never bounce or force. To do so puts tiny tears in muscles and tendons. Though you may feel little from them now, they provide the scar tissue and rough spots for mineral crystallization that will plague you in later years.

Don't be confused by the huge array of exercise books making conflicting claims for the supremacy for their systems. The main trick in exercise is not the particular movements but *the doing*. Most people don't do it daily. And when they do, they strain. Never strain. Anytime you ache the next day, you are going too hard. The body does not need to be inflamed in order to improve. Inflammation is counterproductive.

For the cardiovascular system—walk. It is the simplest, best exercise there is. Thirty minutes a day is the minimum. If you are keen—jog. With a year of optimum nutrition and exercise you will be vastly improved. You may pay a bit of puff to get a high-performance body. But once you have, the little exercise it takes to keep it is one of life's great bargains.

Do Vitamins Improve Athletic Performance?

Most athletes take vitamin and mineral supplements. At the University of Auckland we couldn't find a single one who had not used them. In fact, 84 percent of Olympic athletes use supplements.[2] Well-known coaches such as D. Talbot of Canada believe that success is not possible without them.[3]

When we started to study the effects of vitamins on physical performance in 1975, over 90 percent of the athletes recruited for our studies already used supplements. Everyone took them in a haphazard manner based on hearsay, casual reading and advice from other athletes and coaches. Not one had done any measurements of his possible individual needs. Not one knew which were the essential vitamins and minerals, or which ones were likely to be deficient in his diet or which were likely to be needed in greater quantities for athletics.

In addition, many of the athletes were taking all sorts of weird concoctions, including bee pollen, royal jelly, apple-cider vinegar, Russian "ginseng" (a common Siberian weed), digestive enzymes, DMSO (di-methyl sulphoxide), aloe vera, procaine, various animal-gland extracts and "Vitamin B_{15}."[4] There is no scientific evidence that any of these substances improve athletic performance. No wonder some athletes swear by supplements while others swear *at* them.

Although supplements have always been popular with athletes, few good studies have been done to test them. Vague advice abounds. In their authoritative text *Modern Principles of Athletic Training,* Klafs and Arnheim state that endurance events may increase the need for Vitamin B complex and Vitamin C as much as fifteen times. But they give no actual amounts to multiply by fifteen, nor any evidence for their statement.[5] As we have seen, the B complex is a series of different vitamins, each needed in different amounts with wide individual variations in requirements. Taking an arbitrary combination is very unlikely to improve performance. Indeed, taking fifteen times the current RDA of 18 mg for niacin before a race might slow you down. With or without other B vitamins, 270 mg of niacin causes a skin flush and a prickle that feels like a quick broil from the inside.

Research on the use of vitamins in athletics is very fragmentary. It has been known for fifty years, for instance, that requirements for Vitamin B_1 (thiamine) increase with high energy expenditure and with high carbohydrate intake, both usual in athletics. This vitamin is used continuously in sugar metabolism.[6] Consequently, some athletes believe that extra B_1 inhibits fatigue in endurance events. Winning Australian Olympic athletes do have higher thiamine intakes than losing athletes.[7] But it is impossible to prove a cause-and-effect relationship by studying thiamine alone. As we have seen, like all B vitamins, thiamine operates only in *synergy* with the rest of the nutrient complex. The same goes for B_3 and B_{12}, both used a lot by athletes. With much scientific ado about nothing, silly single-nutrient studies have shown that neither B_3 nor B_{12} has any effect on strength or endurance.[8]

Vitamin C is a bit different. Its hundreds of functions in the exercising body[9] make it less of a scientific sin to study it alone. Extra C before competition may offer a marginal advantage in endurance events, because body stores of C are depleted rapidly by exercise.[10] Extra C may also increase adrenaline during exercise.[11] It also helps the body use free fats as an energy source, thereby saving glycogen, which might improve endurance performance.[12] Loading up on C before a competition may also benefit oxygen metabolism directly.[13] Again, all these actions are no good by themselves. Other parts of the energy production cycle require at least the entire Vitamin B complex and probably A, D and E in order to function adequately.[14] Without a considerable quantity of these complementary vitamins, the extra C may be unusable.

Most of the single-nutrient studies also err by looking for short-term stimulant effects on performance. Many participants in these experiments have used the supplements for only a few days or weeks.[15] As we have seen, the real purpose of nutrient supplements is to build a better body. Because of the principle of physiological dynamics, requiring the turnover of generations of cells, this process is slow. Deficiency studies provide excellent examples of the time scale involved. Diets very deficient in Vitamin C, for instance, reduce blood C levels almost to nil within three weeks. It takes eighteen weeks, however, for enough cells to die and new, defective cells to grow, before the first degenerative signs of scurvy begin to appear.[16]

At the healthy end of the scale, supplemental nutrients may take even longer to show benefits. A big plus in athletic performance is efficient use of oxygen, which depends on how much blood you have and how many red (oxygen-carrying) cells it contains. Good nutrition and regular training can increase both blood volume and red blood cells by 25 percent.[17] With the help of Vitamin C, new capillaries grow in the heart and skeletal muscles to carry the improved blood,[18] and there is a huge improvement in performance. But the whole process may take five years. Between three and six months is the absolute minimum period before you can expect a nutrition effect to show in athletics. Studies of supplementation of athletes over a few days or weeks are useless.

Complete Supplements Do Improve Performance

Multiple vitamin and mineral supplements form an essential part of the diet of Soviet Olympic athletes,[19] although we hear little about it in the West. World-renowned running coach Arthur Lydiard is one of the few Westerners who have real access to Soviet sports medicine. He has told me numerous times how extensively East German coaches have used multiple nutrient supplements in the last decade. During the same period their athletes have gained world supremacy.

But until we began in 1975 at the University of Auckland, studies in Western society were virtually nonexistent. First we studied long-distance runners, to test supplement effects on endurance performance. From pilot studies, we had already designed a system of analysis which contained measures of dietary, medical, physiological, biochemical and behavioral variables. We formed these into a matrix and spent two years inventing a computer program to solve it and relate physical variables to nutrient requirements. Most of the nutrients we used are listed in

Table 7. With the program we can determine a suitable individual supplement, monitor its effects and evaluate changes in physiology and performance.

We also measured levels of toxic metals and other pollutants in the body, with the aim of eliminating them. We were especially concerned to eliminate arsenic, mercury, lead, cadmium, aluminum and excessive copper. Because of food and environmental pollution, most of us have too much of these substances in our bodies. As we saw in Chapter 3, excessive levels cause physical and mental disorders. No one has examined their effects on athletic performance, but it's a safe bet they are detrimental.

Our first study used four experienced male marathon runners aged twenty-six to thirty-five. We divided them into two groups of two, matched for age, marathon experience, previous marathon times and stage of training. Then we designed an individual vitamin and mineral supplement for each. The four athletes were randomly assigned to one of the two groups. In the first group each athlete received his individual vitamin and mineral supplement; in the second group each received a daily placebo that looked and tasted like the real supplement but contained no vitamins or minerals. For six months supplements and placebos were handed out in envelopes of one-month supplies, containing thirty or thirty-one daily packs. The athletes were instructed to take them at the main meal of the day. The study was a "double-blind," that is, neither we nor the runners knew who was getting the real supplements. At the three-month point the code was switched so that those who had been receiving the placebos now received the real vitamins and minerals and vice versa. Throughout the experiment none of the athletes were given any indication that placebos were being used. At the debriefing afterward, all believed that they had been receiving real supplements throughout.

We tested improvements over twenty-mile training runs or marathon races run during the six-month period. The results are shown in Figure 3. Their times were considerably better when

Table 7: Major Vitamins and Minerals Used for Supplements*

Substance	*U.S. RDA (1980)*	*Range for Normal Nutrition (per day)*	*Range for Treatment of Deficiency (per day)*
Vitamin A	800–1,000 mcgRE†	1,000–6,000 mcgRE†	1,000–20,000 mcgRE†
Vitamin B_1 (thiamine)	1.0–1.5 mg	2–75 mg	50–600 mg
Vitamin B_2 (riboflavine)	1.2–1.7 mg	2–55 mg	50–150 mg
Vitamin B_3 (niacin)	13–19 mg	20–150 mg	100–1,000 mg
Vitamin B_5 (pantothenic acid)		10–50 mg	50–200
Vitamin B_6 (pyridoxine)	2.0–2.2 mg	10–75 mg	50–300 mg
Vitamin B_{12} (cyanocobalamin)	3 mcg	10–100 mcg	100–300 mcg
Folic acid	400 mcg	0.5–2.0 mg	3–30 mg
Biotin		2.0–5.0 mg	5–100 mg
Inositol		100–500 mg	100–1,000 mg
Para-amino-benzoic Acid		50–100 mg	100–500 mg
Choline		100–300 mg	200–2,000 mg
Vitamin C	45 mg	500–2,000 mg	2,000–8,000 mg
Vitamin D	5–10 mcg‡	5–50 mcg‡	50–250 mcg‡
Vitamin E	8–10 TE§	50–600 TE§	600–1,200 TE§
Zinc	15 mg	15–50 mg	50–150 mg
Iron	10–18 mg	20–30 mg	30–50 mg
Calcium	800–1,200 mg	800–1,200 mg	1,000–3,500 mg
Magnesium	300–400 mg	400–1,000 mg	1,000–2,000 mg
Manganese		10–50 mg	50–100 mg
Phosphorus	800–1,200 mg	800–1,500 mg	1,000–2,000 mg
Potassium		1,000–3,500 mg	1,000–5,000 mg
Copper		0.5–2.0 mg	2–5 mg
Molybdenum		10–150 mcg	50–500 mcg
Chromium		0.2–0.5 mg	0.5–2.0 mg
Selenium		50–150 mcg	0.5–2.0 mg
Iodine	150 mcg	100–250 mcg	100–600 mcg

* Essential amino acids and other nutrient substances are used also, but are beyond the scope of discussion here. Sulfur, tin, silcion, vanadium, cobalt and nickel are not included, as suitable supplement forms are not available in the United States. Fluorine is usually available in the water supply.

† RE = retinol equivalents, the new way of expressing Vitamin A activity.

‡ Vitamin D is now expressed as mcg cholecalciferol activity.

§ TE = alpha-tocopherol equivalents, the new way of expressing Vitamin E activity.

Figure 3: Seconds-per-mile improvement in time trials or races of 20+ miles (including marathons) for four experienced marathon runners with and without supplementation

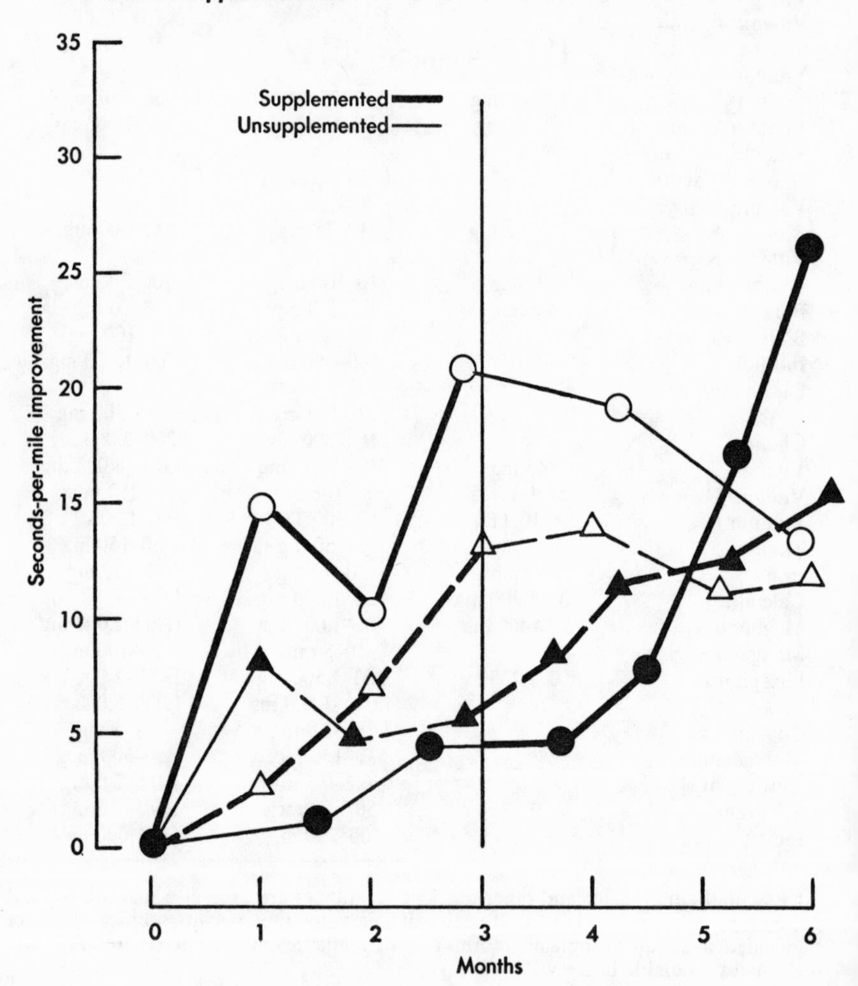

the athletes were receiving the real vitamins and minerals. The best runner improved his marathon time by two minutes eight seconds in the three months with placebos. With real supplements in the second three months, he improved a further eight minutes fifty-two seconds, a significant advance. Both runners who received real supplements during the first three months improved rapidly during that time. When their supplements were switched to placebos in the second three months, performance fell off for one and did not improve for the other. The two runners who got the real supplements during the second three months overtook the other two whose supplements had been replaced by placebos during that period. So, even though three months of supplementation is really too short, results suggest a definite effect in improving endurance performance.

In a second study we examined the effects of supplements on strength. We took four experienced weight lifters and divided them into two groups of two, matched for age, weightlifting ability and stage of training. We devised two special strength tests for the experiment. In the first of these tests the athlete laid his weaker arm on a board slanted down at 35° and raised a dumbbell clasped in his fist with the palm facing upward, while maintaining full contact with the board with the upper arm. In the second test the athlete lay with head uppermost on a board slanted at 35°. A weight was then strapped to his feet and he had to raise the weight with his legs straight until it was above his head. We also measured performance at the Olympic lifts, the press, where the weight is pushed above the head by the strength of the arms alone, and the clean and jerk, where the athlete can bend his legs and use a sudden jerk to get the weight aloft. We didn't measure the Olympic snatch, where the weight is snatched above the head right from the ground, because this lift depends more heavily on speed and technique. We were measuring strength.

The study proceeded with controls like the first one for six months. The results of the special strength tests are shown in Figure 4. The two lifters who took supplements the first three

Figure 4: Combined percentage increase in maximum poundage used in special exercises for four experienced weight lifters with and without supplementation

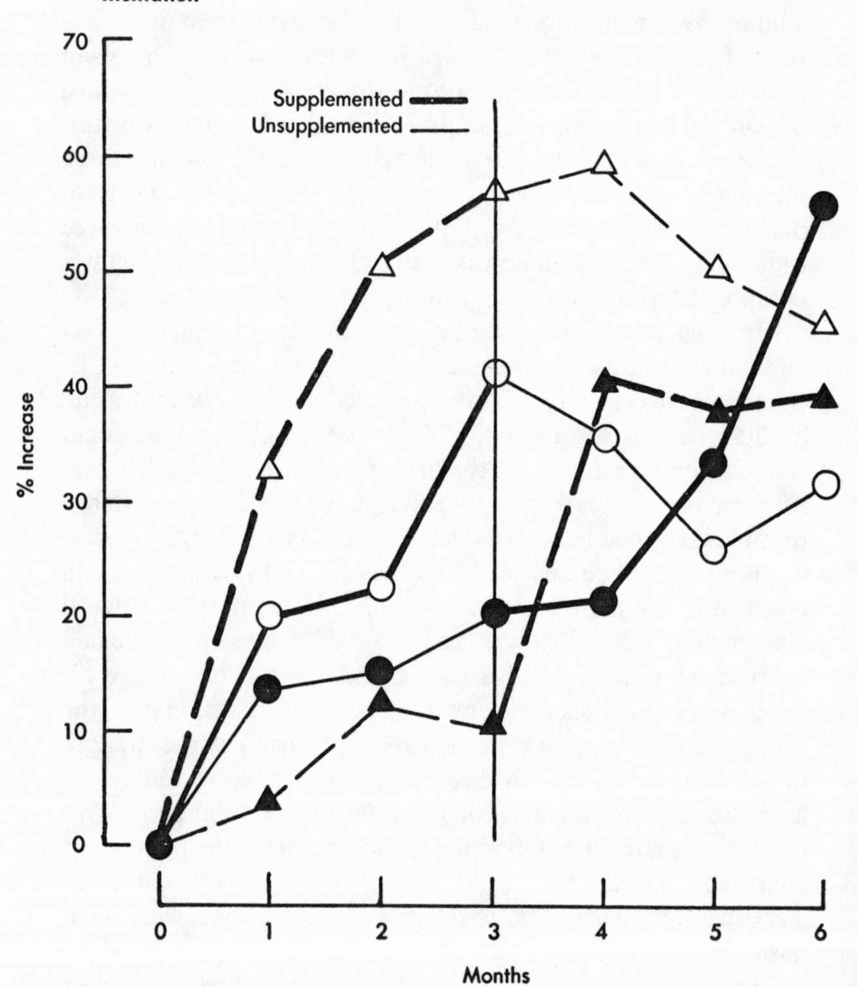

months increased their strength very quickly in both these exercises. At the end of three months one had increased his strength by nearly 60 percent and the other by over 40 percent. The two lifters who had taken placebos the first three months showed a much smaller increase (10–20 percent). During the second three months, however, when their placebos were changed to real supplements, they caught up with the first two weight lifters, whose performance slumped when they were taken off the active supplements.

Performances at the Olympic lifts increased also. Figure 5 shows that the combined increase in poundage for the press and the clean and jerk was 8 percent and 4 percent for the two lifters who took the supplements during the first three months. The unsupplemented lifters showed very little improvement during that period. When put on supplements, however, during the second three months they both increased performance about 4 percent. Improvements of 4 percent to 8 percent don't sound huge, but these men were near the limits of strength before the studies began. Translated into weights, the improvements were between thirty-six and seventy-four pounds, enough to raise a top lifter from ignominy to a gold medal.

Encouraged by the results of these two studies, I designed a better one. I divided ten experienced male marathon runners, whose best times were between two and a half and three hours, into two groups of five. They were matched in pairs for age, marathon experience, previous marathon times and stage of training. All had run at least six marathons. I randomly assigned them to either an experimental group getting the real supplements or a control group getting the placebos. For twenty-six weeks the supplements and placebos were given out as for the other studies, except that the packs now contained twenty-eight days of daily supplements. Every four weeks we measured heart rate, temperature, blood pressure and a whole range of blood variables, such as you would have taken in an annual physical. Improvements in performance were measured by twenty-mile time trials or marathon races.

Figure 5: ***Percentage increases in poundage used in press and clean and jerk combined for four experienced weight lifters, with and without supplementation***

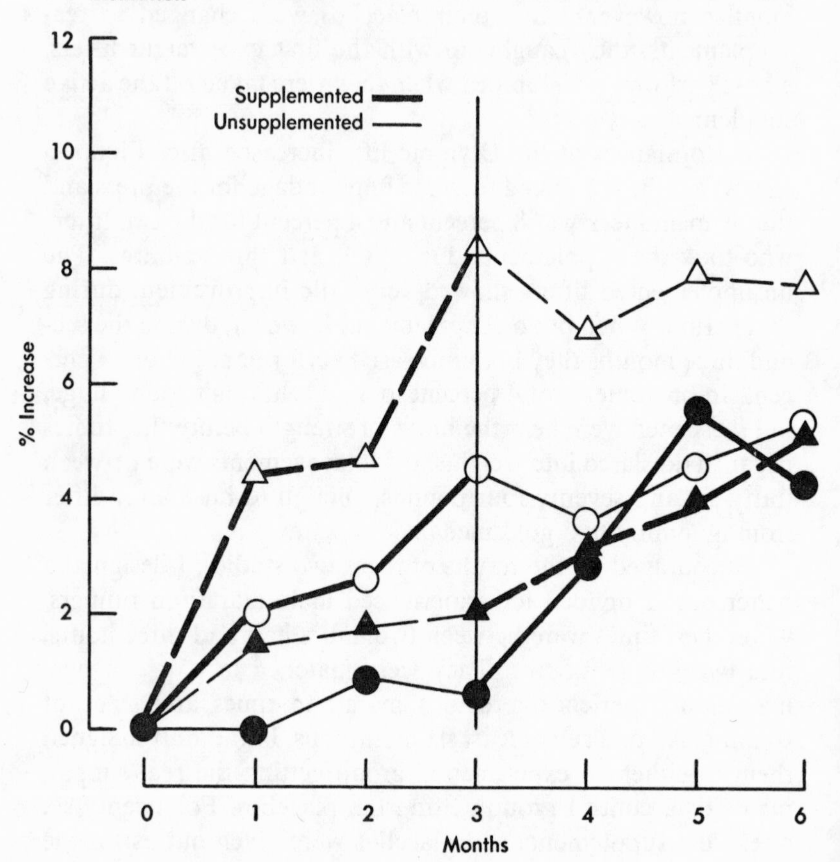

Table 8 lists the details and resulting improvements. Figure 6 shows performance over the six months for each group. This figure also shows the mean marathon improvements of the groups in the twelve months prior to the study. The runners taking supplements made big improvements in marathon time: from 9 minutes 44 seconds to *28 minutes 25 seconds.* As a result of continued training, three of the men taking placebos improved also, as you might expect from their training, but by much less (7 minutes 1 second to 11 minutes 20 seconds). The difference between the groups was a significant eleven-minute superiority in the supplemented group. In the marathon race used as a test,

Table 8: Comparison Data for the Two Marathon Groups

Subjects	*Age*	*No. of Previous Marathons or 20+-mile races*	*Best Marathon Time*	*Marathon Time at Conclusion of Study*	*Improvement*
EXPERIMENTAL GROUP			HOURS/MINS/SECS	HOURS/MINS/SECS	MINS/SECS
E1	28	7	2 : 31 : 40	2 : 21 : 56	9 : 44
E2	30	18	2 : 53 : 20	2 : 38 : 02	17 : 18
E3	38	6	2 : 59 : 17	2 : 30 : 52	28 : 25
E4	44	25	2 : 48 : 01	2 : 33 : 31	15 : 30
				MEAN IMPROVEMENT	17 : 44
CONTROL GROUP					
C1	29	6	2 : 36 : 18	2 : 27 : 48	8 : 30
C2	32	9	2 : 52 : 00	2 : 57 : 03	(−5 : 03)
C3	35	11	2 : 55 : 23	2 : 48 : 22	7 : 01
C4	42	19	2 : 50 : 35	2 : 39 : 15	11 : 20
				MEAN IMPROVEMENT (taking C2 as zero)	6 : 43

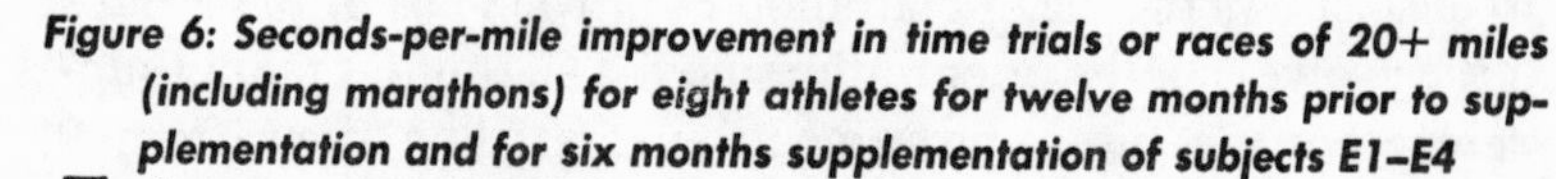

Figure 6: Seconds-per-mile improvement in time trials or races of 20+ miles (including marathons) for eight athletes for twelve months prior to supplementation and for six months supplementation of subjects E1–E4

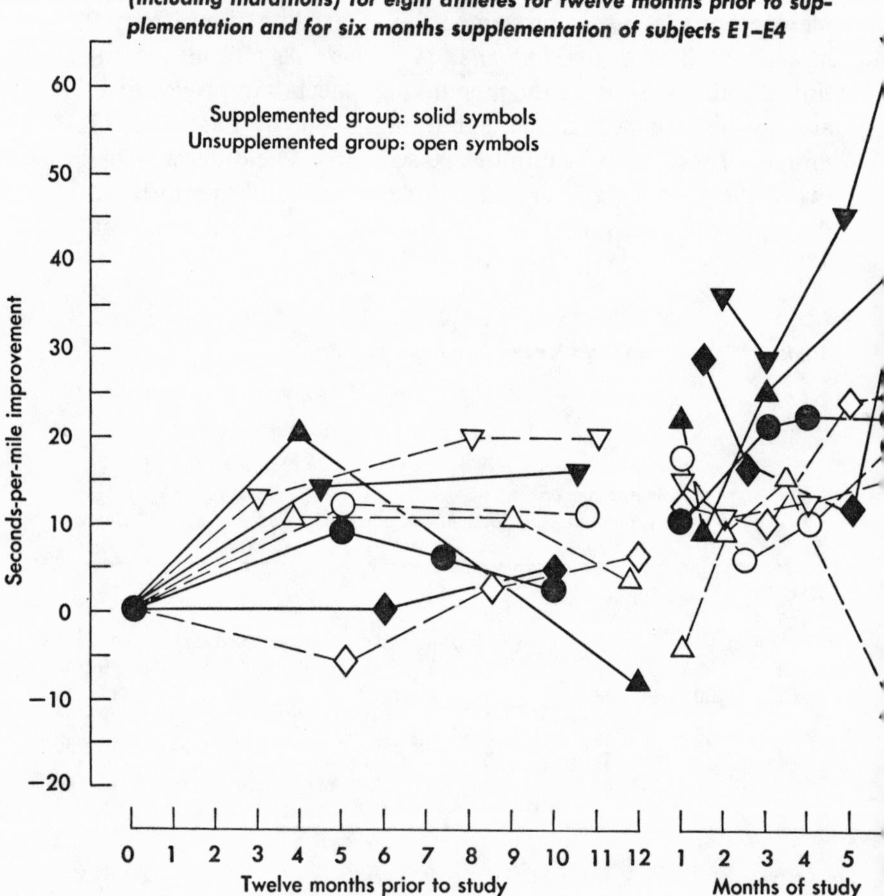

they beat the pants off the placebo group, and a lot of other surprised runners. At the debriefing six runners (three from each group) said they believed active vitamins and minerals were being used throughout. Two expressed doubts but were unable to identify any period when they thought placebos were being used. So placebo effects (that is, effects caused by the *idea* of being in a prestigious study or by taking the supplements, or by the enthusiasm of the scientists) can be ruled out. The result is especially significant considering the ages of the subjects (twenty-eight to forty-four years), when you would expect a decline in athletic performance. Also they showed much lesser rates of improvement over the previous twelve months.

In the course of this experiment, physiological changes occurred in the athletes also. All of the athletes receiving real supplements had their already low resting heart rates (47–55 beats per minute) drop further by an average of 9.1 beats per minute. The heart rates of those on placebos did not change significantly. Resting blood pressures of all those on supplements also dropped reliably, although their pressures were at the lower end of the normal range already.

Their cholesterol levels were also lower than average before the study. Over the six months they dropped further for three of the athletes who were given real supplements. Other beneficial changes occurred too, but the heart rate, blood pressure and cholesterol level changes are the most clearly beneficial because recent studies show that the top half of what are commonly taken as the normal ranges in fact are indicative of widespread cardiovascular disorder in American society.[20] Athletes given placebos showed no such improvements.

In addition, the supplemented athletes had 35 percent fewer minor injuries (fifty-two as opposed to seventy) and 81 percent fewer infections (six as opposed to twenty-eight) than those on placebos. The supplements not only improved performance, but very likely exerted a protective effect upon the body as well. The three types of measurements—improved performance, improved biochemistry and reduced illness and injury—all point to a decided advantage for those taking individual vitamin and mineral supplements. In top competition, where the edge on opponents is often very small, this advantage might make the difference between losing or setting a world record.

In all three of the studies described, the supplemented athletes improved their performances substantially. In the first two experiments the supplementation period was only three months. In the third it was six months. Even so, Figure 6 shows that performance was still improving at the end of this period. We know now that six months is too short a time to test the effects of supplements. Twelve months is more realistic for the physiological changes to occur that raise an athlete from merely good to first class. We are now doing that year-long study at Rockefeller University.

You don't have to be an athlete to benefit from supplements. Give your body even a minimal exercise habit, along with the vitamins and minerals, and it will respond beautifully. We have applied this practice to more than five hundred cases since 1973. The only failures were those people who wanted instant solutions. Like instant coffee, "instant" vitamins are successful only on television commercials. Physiological adaptation is slow. Many people have been on our program of individual supplements now for five to eight years. They are changed men and women. As individual case histories, these records don't carry much scientific clout, because they lack the controlled measurements described in the above studies. Perhaps the effects can best be summed up in the words of one extremely successful young man who has been using our system since 1974. "These days I have only one prayer. Never let me be again the way I was before."

Improved Intelligence

Individual vitamin and mineral supplements also improve mental performance. By 1970 the number of American children with serious problems in their vision, hearing, speech, and mental functioning or emotional reactions was 9,649,000.[21] By 1980 one in every five of our children had some learning disability.[22] Despite alarmist speculation, this has little to do with the slightly increased risk of the trend to have children later in life. There is little doubt that these shocking statistics are related to malnutrition and bodily pollution of the mother and baby. They are doubly bad when we see that the percentage of handicapped children is increasing while the American birth rate is *declining.*

The real tragedy is that much of this suffering is preventable even after birth. Many learning disabilities respond favorably to simple changes in nutrition and simple elimination of pollutants from the child's environment. In my private clinic in New Zealand and in the University of Auckland Psychology Clinic, from 1977 to 1979 I treated sixteen cases of children classified as minimally brain damaged (MBD), hyperactive or slow learner, plus one case of child autism. All were given individually designed vitamin and mineral supplements. All these children had been treated elsewhere without success. Some were found to have toxic metals in their bodies and some had substantial allergies. These were dealt with also. Diets were changed to reduce processed foods, candies and soft drinks. Over periods from three to six months, *every case* showed improvements in behavior, at home, at school and in the clinic, and in motor coordination, speech articulation and reading skills. Some improvements might be expected, because we were using the Stott reading programs from Guelph University in Canada plus our own behavior-modification system to bring them about. We patted each other on the back for our success where other clinics had failed.

What we did not expect were improvements in intelligence quotients. As a matter of course, each child was given Form A of a standardized intelligence test some time after the beginning of treatment and Form B at the end of his time at the clinic. Some were given Form B first, then Form A. We found improvements *between 5 and 35 IQ points* with an average improvement of 17.9 points. When these results first occurred, we thought they might be due to the children becoming more friendly, relaxed and motivated over the course of treatment with our very skilled therapists. So we checked back to cases where no supplements had been used. These showed no significant changes in IQ. We found also that the children who took supplements made significantly bigger gains in reading skills than the children who did not take supplements. They showed greater improvements in behavior too, rated independently by parents, teachers and therapists. The improvements were especially noticeable in emotional reactions. Finally, we could not ignore the evidence. We were convinced. Nutritional changes were the significant variable. They were making the children more intelligent and more emotionally stable.

To the scientific community these case-study results are suggestive but not definitive. But supportive studies have been accumulating in America since the early 1970's. In 1973 Dr. Bernard Rimland, director of the Institute for Child Behavior Research in San Diego, used a formula of B complex, plus extra B_5 and B_6, plus Vitamin C and iron to help emotionally disturbed children. The only individual variable he was able to consider in designing the formulae was the child's body weight. Nevertheless, out of 190 severely disturbed children, 164 showed some improvement over 90 days.[23]

Since then, there have been numerous American studies confirming the beneficial effects of supplements in treating autism[24] and hyperactivity.[25] Dr. Rimland now advocates the use of a vitamin and mineral supplement which is in powder form and therefore excellent for use with children, as it can be mixed with juice or cereal. This formula contains most of the essential vitamins and minerals.[26] Dr. Rimland also emphasizes the removal of toxic metals and other bodily pollutants, and avoidance of "junk" foods, which contain many potentially harmful pollutants in the form of chemical additives. These nonfoods may also contain caffeine, as well as excess starch, sugar and salt.[27] In this connection it is encouraging that in January 1982 the National Institutes of Health declared that, despite the absence of good controlled studies, physicians could try the Feingold additive-free diets for child hyperactivity. One component of this affliction is learning disability.[28]

The studies above show that individual vitamins and minerals improve learning, behavior and emotions. An important recent study confirms our own data that they also improve intelligence. In 1980 Dr. Ruth Harrell and her colleagues at Old Dominion University, Virginia, gave comprehensive vitamin and mineral supplements to a group of five mentally retarded children. Eleven other retarded children received a placebo. Over a period of only four months, the supplemented children increased their IQs by 5.0 to 9.6 points. The unsupplemented children showed no significant change. Over a further four months all sixteen children were given the supplements. The previously unsupplemented group showed an average increase in IQ of 10.2 points with a range of 3 to 21 points. Three of the five children supplemented throughout showed further IQ gains in the second four months. Over the eight months they gained 9, 16 and 25 IQ points respectively.[29] These gains are highly significant, especially as they were achieved with a mixture of different retardation syndromes, including Down's syndrome.

It was not possible for Dr. Harrell to do an individual analysis of each child's nutritional needs. Because of this, the study has been criticized by the American Academy of Pediatrics for the arbitrary nature of the vitamin/mineral formula.[30] Our whole research effort over nine years has been directed at overcoming this problem. It is no easy task. To design an individual supplement for a normal child is frighteningly complex, let alone for a retarded child. Dr. Harrell is to be applauded for her courageous and successful work.

The Academy of Pediatrics also expressed doubt that vitamins and minerals could be used therapeutically with an affliction as diverse as mental retardation, which can be a result of infections, intoxication, trauma, loss of oxygen to the brain or genetic abnormalities. But nutrition knows no boundaries of disease. It improves the functioning of the whole body. So it should benefit just such a wide range of syndromes. The evidence is strong enough to indicate that children who have learning problems should, as standard practice, have evaluations of their nutritional status and bodily pollutants by physicians *competently trained* in nutrition.

Children don't have to be retarded or learning disabled to benefit from vitamins and minerals. In one study in Norfolk, Virginia, children born to mothers who had received extra nutrients during pregnancy had higher IQs than children of mothers who did not.[31] Yet the supplement contained only Vitamins B_1, B_2, B_3 and iron, and the children were tested three to four years later. That even a poor supplement given to the *mothers* could have such long-range effects on their infants indicates the potential power of optimal nutrition. Another study compared poorly nourished black children to a matched group of well-nourished black children over a period of seven years. Each time IQs were tested, the poorly nourished group was between fifteen and twenty IQ points below the other group. At the final testing at age eight, the well-nourished group was twenty-three IQ points above the children who had remained malnourished.[32]

Both of these studies, and Dr. Harrell's work and my own, used standardized intelligence tests. Although these tests have been the subject of controversy in recent years, in February 1982 the National Academy of Sciences finally determined that they are valid measures of intellectual ability.[33] Differences of over twenty IQ points were found in all studies. At the bottom of the scale this is the difference between normalcy and idiocy. At the top of the scale it is the difference between average and exceptionally bright. Clearly, good nutrition can convey a profound intellectual advantage.

Enhanced Memory

There is one universal trait characteristic of our top minds—an excellent memory. A single thermonuclear explosion over key cities would destroy the American economy not only because of the human carnage, but because the electromagnetic fields created would erase the memories of government, business and health computers. The same can occur with human brains; a single blow can erase previous memory. Like the computer, however, the human brain's ability to relearn and store new memories is usually left undamaged. This is not what happens in the slow degeneration of the brain that results from poor nutrition. The brain still loses some old memories but, more important, the ability to learn and retain new material is progressively damaged. For example, the unfortunate victims of Alzheimer's disease (premature senility) are often completely helpless because they cannot remember even for five minutes where they are or what they are doing. Less severe but still unpleasant is the gradual loss of memory function that begins to occur after age forty in many otherwise apparently healthy people.

Yet some people retain a clear memory until death. One reason is a healthy cardiovascular system, which ensures a constant supply of blood to the brain. The other reason is good nutrition, which supplies the brain cells with adequate nutrients and prevents them from being poisoned by toxic metals or other pullutants. We are beginning to learn just how sensitive memory is to nutrition. One pertinent example is choline, a dietary cofactor of the B complex.

Choline may affect memory because it enhances brain acetylcholine, a brain-transmitter substance necessary for the passage of impulses from one nerve to another. Various drugs which enhance the quantity or activity of brain acetylcholine improve memory, even in rats.[34] They work in humans too. Dr. Kenneth Davis and his colleagues at the Palo Alto VA Hospital in California gave nineteen healthy young men with normal memories injections of physostigmine, a drug known to stimulate acetylcholine activity. For a while the men developed supermemories.[35] Physostigmine has the same memory-enhancing effect in elderly people.[36] Ribonucleic acid (RNA), that essential constitutent of every human cell, which is plentiful in fish and yeast, also improves memory above normal in rats,[37] again probably because it stimulates acetylcholine activity. So there is *some* basis to the belief that fish is food for the brain.

Even choline itself works. In 1978 Dr. N. Sitaram and his colleagues gave arecholine to young adults with normal memories (mean age twenty-three). For a while long-term memory improved significantly. In a second experiment they gave young men ten grams of simple choline chloride. Again, long-term memory was temporarily improved.[38] Unfortunately, it does not work for everyone. Memory is far more complex than a mere function of acetylcholine activity. Multiple nutrient interactions are essential. If a choline supplement alone has an effect, it can do so only by drawing complementary nutrients from the diet or from other parts of the body. This is one likely reason why these studies work better on young healthy people, whose bodies probably contain the necessary nutrients in quantity, rather than on the elderly, who may have multiple nutrient deficiencies. Nevertheless, if arbitrary amounts of choline alone can enhance a complex mental function like human memory *at all,* consider what a complete, individual supplement might do over a long period.

The practice of enhancing physical and mental performance by improving nutrition is not yet widespread. It will be. It is not very difficult even now. In the closing years of this century the streamlining of systems of individual nutritional analysis will make them widely available. When this happens, our present conceptions of the limits of human capacity will become obsolete. Until now, humanity has survived, albeit sickly, on less than adequate nutrition. But recently we have discovered how to use computers to design individual supplements that produce better nutrition than the human organism has ever experienced before. I and my colleagues have spent the last ten years establishing what we believe is the most advanced of these systems. When widely applied, their beneficial effects on strength, endurance, intelligence, memory and emotions will produce better human beings than ever before in history.

CHAPTER 6

YOUR INDIVIDUAL BIOCHEMICAL EQUATION

THE *flesh* IS ALWAYS WILLING. Only the spirit is weak. The greatest barrier to improving your nutrition is habit. Changing your diet, avoiding pollutants, even taking vitamins and minerals regularly are difficult tasks. In a society of instant everything, we are conditioned to expect immediate success. But the body conforms to immutable laws of physiological dynamics, not to the dictates of Madison Avenue. Adaptation is slow. Unless you are determined to stay on a supplement program for at least six months, don't start.

If you do adopt the advice in this book, your body will still be changing two years later. It must have time for cell turnover. The successive generations of improved cells each need three to five months to grow and mature. Just like a neglected plant which is then given a rich nutrient mixture, you have to wait for new foliage growth to see real improvement.

Also, if you want the ultimate benefit, you must challenge your body with progressive exercise, no matter if you begin only by swinging your arms ten times as you get out of bed. The body will respond magnificently. If you include progressive exercise in your health program, your body may go on changing and improving for a *decade.*

Before you begin calculating your supplement, look at Figure 7. It gives a general picture of each individual's need for each essential nutrient. A certain level of deficiency of a nutrient, shown by the shaded area on the left-hand side, eventually causes death. Above that level, the body functions marginally for a wide range of low intake of any single nutrient, although

Figure 7: Degree of optimal bodily function with differing amounts of a nutrient

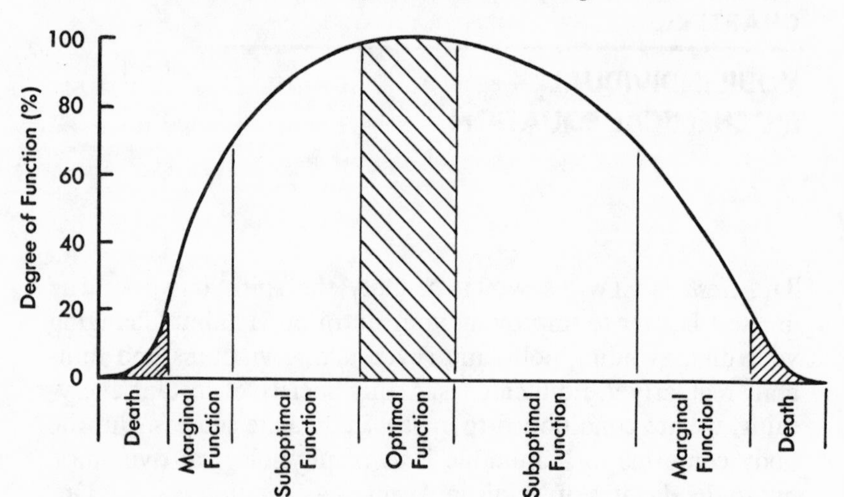

you may not show any overt illness. Then there is a wide range of supply that gives reasonable but still suboptimal function. Then there is a narrow band where intake of a particular nutrient is optimal and provides exactly the right amounts for its interactions with other nutrients. Then there is a wide range of oversupply, which again causes suboptimal bodily function and a further range where function declines to marginal. These are wider than the range for undersupply, because most vitamins and minerals are low in toxicity. Finally, there is a range of toxic oversupply which so interferes with normal function that it causes death.

There have been a few cases of fatal poisoning from huge overdoses of the fat-soluble Vitamins A and D and the mineral selenium, but not with any other nutrients. Nevertheless, every nutrient can be toxic if taken in excess. When filling out the questionnaire, don't add any unnecessary nutrients "just in case." Stick to the questions that describe *you.*

Remember, the formula is not final. As your body adapts to improve its functions, eliminate deficiencies and use the nutrients more efficiently, requirements change also. We are only just learning how the amount of a vitamin used by the cells changes bodily demands for that nutrient and influences the production of enzymes which enable it to be absorbed and utilized by the body. When supplements are taken over a long period, in conjunction with exercise to stimulate the building of higher performance cells, the nature of the organism changes. Its muscular, vascular, glandular and nervous tissues improve in both structure and function, and there is a gradual beneficial shift in the whole spectrum of enzyme chemistry. We don't know much about it yet except that requirements for optimum nutrition may be radically altered. So retest yourself periodically for at least eighteen months and adjust your formula to suit.

Table 9 lists the essential vitamins and minerals for which requirements can be assessed in this self-help system. The lines following the BASIC FORMULA for each nutrient are for putting in the additions as you answer the questions. You can do this exercise best by copying the table onto squared paper.

Do not use the final formula until you have read Chapter 7. Chapter 7 contains important modifications that must be made before you use the formula. Remember, you use the formula at your own discretion and sole risk. Please also remember that this assessment is not for people suffering from disease. It is not a prescription and does not purport to treat any illness. It should not be used in place of medical treatment. If you are ill, go to a physican competently trained in nutrition. If you are below eighteen years of age, the BASIC FORMULA in Table 9 can be used freely. Formulae built upon it, by using the questionnaire, should be referred to a physician competently trained in nutrition before being used with children. Nutrient demands during growth differ considerably from those in adulthood. The same applies during pregnancy and lactation. The nutrient demands of the growing fetus and suckling infant change the mother's nutrient needs enormously. If you are pregnant, see an obstetrician competently trained in nutrition.

Table 9: Formula Calculations

	Basic Formula	
Vitamin A	2,000 IU	
Vitamin B_1	10 mg	
Vitamin B_2	10 mg	
Vitamin B_3	50 mg	
Vitamin B_5	20 mg	
Vitamin B_6	20 mg	
Vitamin B_{12}	20 mcg	
Folic acid	200 mcg	
Biotin	500 mcg	
Choline	100 mg	
Inositol	100 mg	
PABA	50 mg	
Vitamin C	1,000 mg	
Bioflavonoids	100 mg	
Vitamin D	200 IU	
Vitamin E	200 IU	
Calcium	500 mg	
Magnesium	250 mg	
Phosphorus	200 mg	
Potassium	25 mg	
Iron	10 mg	
Copper	1 mg	
Zinc	5 mg	
Manganese	5 mg	
Molybdenum	50 mcg	
Chromium	25 mcg	
Selenium	25 mcg	
Iodine	50 mcg	
Lysine	These nutrients may be required depending on answers to questions.	
Linoleic acid		
Pectin		
Digestive enzymes		
Lecithin		

THE BASIC FORMULA

1. Weight

☐ If you weigh 120 lbs or less, start the questionnaire with the BASIC FORMULA shown in Table 9.

☐ For weights 121–180 lbs, increase all items in the BASIC FORMULA by half (e.g., Vitamin A 2,000 IU becomes Vitamin A 3,000 IU).

☐ For weights above 180 lbs, double the BASIC FORMULA.

2. Overweight

☐ Ideal for height: Gold Star

☐ Up to 20 lb above ideal: O.K.

☐ 20–40 lb above ideal:

Increase Vitamin C 500 mg. Increase the porportion of high-fiber foods: whole grain breads, brown rice, raw vegetables.

☐ More than 40 lb overweight:

Increase Vitamin C 1,000 mg. Increase high-fiber foods. Read Chapter 8 on obesity.

3. Home location

☐ If you live in a major city or near an industrial area:

Increase Vitamin A 2,000 IU; C 1,000 mg; bioflavonoids 100 mg; E 100 IU; zinc 10 mg; selenium 50 mcg.

4. Smoking

☐ Nonsmoker: Gold Star

☐ Exposed to smokers most of working day (i.e., involuntary smoker):

Increase Vitamin C 500 mg; bioflavonoids 50 mg; zinc 5 mg.

☐ Smoke fewer than five cigarettes* daily.
Increase Vitamin A (carotenoid form) 2,000 IU; C 500 mg; bioflavonoids 50 mg; zinc 5 mg.

☐ Smoke five to fifteen cigarettes daily:
Increase Vitamin A (carotenoid form) 4,000 IU; B_1 5 mg; B_2 5 mg; C 750 mg; bioflavonoids 75 mg; zinc 5 mg.

☐ Smoke sixteen to thirty cigarettes daily.
Increase Vitamin A (carotenoid form) 6,000 IU; B_1 10 mg; B_2 10 mg; C 1,000 mg; bioflavonoids 100 mg; zinc 10 mg.

☐ Smoke more than thirty cigarettes daily.
Increase Vitamin A (carotenoid form) 9,000 IU; B_1 10 mg; B_2 10 mg; C 1,500 mg; bioflavonoids 150 mg; zinc 15 mg.

5. Alcohol

☐ Up to two drinks a day:† O.K.

☐ Two to five drinks a day:
Increase Vitamin A 2,000 IU; B_1 50 mg; B_2 25 mg; B_3 100 mg; B_6 20 mg; B_{12} 50 mcg; C 250 mg; bioflavonoids 25 mg; folic acid 100 mcg; magnesium 50 mg; potassium 5 mg; zinc 5 mg.

☐ Six drinks or more a day:
Increase Vitamin A 4,000 IU; B_1 80 mg; B_2 40 mg; B_3 200 mg; B_6 30 mg; folic acid 200 mcg; C 500 mg; bioflavonoids 50 mg; magnesium 100 mg; potassium 10 mg; zinc 10 mg.
Add linoleic acid 800 mg.

6. Processed carbohydrates (starches and sugars, e.g., white bread, pasta, cake, candy, biscuits)

* Pipe smokers: one pipe = two cigarettes. Cigar smokers: one medium-sized cigar = three cigarettes. Regarding nutrient depletion of the body, low-tar or specially filtered cigarettes are *not* safer than others. For "I don't inhale" smokers, don't kid yourself. Everyone inhales, it's continuously necessary for life.

† 1 drink = 1 8-oz glass of beer, 1 3½-oz glass of table wine or 1 oz of hard liquor.

☐ Less than once a week: Gold Star.
☐ Once or twice a week: O.K.
☐ Every day:
Increase Vitamin B_1 30 mg; B_5 20 mg; B_6 10 mg; magnesium 50 mg; potassium 20 mg; manganese 5 mg; chromium 50 mcg.
At most meals:
Increase Vitamin B_1 50 mg; B_5 30 mg; B_6 10 mg; folic acid 100 mcg; magnesium 100 mg; potassium 10 mg; manganese 5 mg; chromium 100 mcg.

7. Saturated fats
☐ As little as possible: Gold Star.
☐ Average (in meat, butter, cheese): O.K.
☐ Enjoy fried foods (e.g., bacon, fried eggs):
Increase Vitamin B_6 5 mg.
☐ Enjoy fatty meats, bologna, sausages, hamburgers:
Increase Vitamin B_6 10 mg; C 250 mg; bioflavonoids 25 mg.
Add lecithin 500 mg.
☐ Prefer fatty foods:
Increase Vitamin B_6 10 mg; C 500 mg; bioflavonoids 50 mg.
Add lecthin 1,000 mg; linoleic acid 400 mg.

8. Preserved or smoked meats (e.g., hamburger, sausages, bologna, canned meats)
☐ Once a week or less: O.K.
☐ Two to four times a week:
Increase Vitamin C 250 mg; bioflavonoids 25 mg; E 50 IU; selenium 25 mcg.
☐ More than four times a week;
Increase Vitamin C 500 mg; bioflavonoids 50 mg; E 100 IU; selenium 50 mcg.

9. Canned food (any kind, including soups, vegetables, meat, fish)

☐ Once a week or less: O.K.
☐ Two to four times a week:
Increase potassium 20 mg; zinc 5 mg.
☐ More than four times a week:
Increase calcium 200 mg; potassium 30 mg; zinc 10 mg.

10. Fresh raw fruit and vegetables (not canned or frozen or cooked vegetables or fruit)
☐ Every day: Gold Star
☐ Two or three times a week:
Increase Vitamin A 1,000 IU; folic acid 50 mcg.
☐ Less than twice a week:
Increase Vitamin A 2,000 IU; folic acid 100 mcg; C 250 mg; bioflavonoids 25 mg.

11. Salt
☐ If you avoid all salt in your diet:
Increase iodine 100 mcg.
☐ If you sprinkle salt on your food *before* tasting it and/or like salty foods:
Increase zinc 10 mg; potassium 25 mg.

12. If you drink more than five cups of coffee, tea, colas or cocoa:
Increase potassium 50 mg.

13. If you eat a high-protein diet:
Increase Vitamin B_6 20 mg; B_{12} 30 mcg; folic acid 100 mcg.

14. If you are losing your sense of taste or smell, or if you prefer highly seasoned foods:
Increase Vitamin A 1,000 IU; zinc 10 mg.

15. On missing a meal, do you feel weakness, tremor, nausea, dizziness, irritability or anxiety? OR do you have to snack

between meals, especially on "junk" food, biscuits, cakes or candy to "keep your strength up"? If so:

Increase Vitamin B_3 50 mg; B_6 20 mg; inositol 500 mg; C 500 mg; bioflavonoids 50 mg; calcium 200 mg; magnesium 100 mg; zinc 10 mg; manganese 5 mg; chromium 100 mcg.

16. If you have a very poor appetite and no physical cause can be found:

Increase Vitamin A 1,000 IU; B_1 5 mg; B_2 5 mg; B_3 20 mg; B_5 20 mg; B_6 5 mg; B_{12} 10 mcg; folic acid 100 mcg; biotin 200 mcg; phosphorus 50 mg; zinc 5 mg.

17. Skin conditions

☐ If you habitually have very dry skin:

Increase Vitamin B_3 50 mg; potassium 25 mg.

☐ If you are unable to suntan or have white spots or white stripes on the pink areas of your fingernails:

Increase Vitamin A 1,000 IU; zinc 30 mg.

☐ If you get recurrent acne:

Increase Vitamin A* 5,000 IU; potassium 30 mg; zinc 30 mg.

Eat eggs, onions and garlic for sulfur.

☐ If you get recurrent mild eczema:

Increase Vitamin A 1,000 IU: B_1 10 mg; B_2 10 mg; B_3 50 mg; B_5 30 mg; B_6 10 mg; B_{12} 50 mcg; folic acid 100 mcg; biotin 200 mcg; inositol 200 mg; iodine 100 mcg.

☐ If you get recurrent mild patches of psoriasis:

Increase Vitamin A 1,000 IU; B_6 40 mg; zinc 45 mg.

Eat eggs, onions and garlic freely for sulfur.

18. If you have weak, brittle fingernails:

Increase Vitamin A 1,000 IU; B_6 10 mg; C 500 mg; bio-

* The best form of Vitamin A for acne is cis retinoic acid (Hoffmann La Roche). If your acne is bad enough so that you are being treated for it by your physician, disregard this question and ask your physician about cis retinoic acid.

flavonoids 50 mg; D 200 IU; calcium 200 mg; magnesium 100 mg; phosphorus 100 mg; iron 5 mg; zinc 10 mg.
Add silicon 100 mg. If you cannot obtain silicon, eat raw vegetables daily for their silicon content.
Eat eggs at least three times weekly and onions and garlic freely for sulfur.

19. Hair conditions

☐ If you have poor hair condition no matter what you try:
Increase Vitamin B_1 10 mg; B_2 10 mg; B_3 20 mg; B_5 15 mg; B_6 10 mg; B_{12} 20 mcg; folic acid 50 mcg; biotin 200 mcg; PABA 100 mg; iodine 50 mcg.

☐ If your hair is prematurely graying or excessively falling out:
Increase Vitamin B_5 50 mg; B_6 10 mg; folic acid 200 mcg; biotin 300 mcg; inositol 100 mg; PABA 100 mg; zinc 20 mg.
Eat eggs, onions and garlic for sulfur.

20. If you have mild allergies to fur, dust, feathers, pollen:
Increase Vitamin B_6 10 mg; potassium 10 mg; zinc 5 mg; manganese 5 mg.

21. If your sexual behavior is *physically* below par, or has declined markedly in recent years and you are less than seventy years old:
Increase Vitamin B_6 30 mg; E 100 IU; zinc 20 mg; selenium 50 mcg; molybdenum 50 mcg.

22. If you tend to get irritable or nervous with little reason:
Increase Vitamin B_1 10 mg; B_2 10 mg; B_3 50 mg; B_5 50 mg; B_6 10 mg; B_{12} 25 mcg; PABA 50 mg; C 250 mg; bioflavonoids 25 mg; D 100 IU; calcium 100 mg; magnesium 100 mg; phosphorus 50 mg.
Avoid caffeine—tea, coffee, cocoa, colas, chocolate.

Most soft drinks contain substantial amounts of caffeine.

23. If you tend to suffer recurrent depressions and no physical cause can be found:
    Increase Vitamin B_1 20 mg; B_2 20 mg; B_3 100 mg; B_5 30 mg; B_6 25 mg; folic acid 100 mcg; C 500 mg; bioflavonoids 50 mg; calcium 200 mg; magnesium 100 mg; zinc 20 mg.

24. If you get recurrent constipation and no physical cause can be found:
    Increase Vitamin B_1 10 mg; B_2 10 mg; B_3 50 mg; B_5 20 mg; B_6 10 mg; B_{12} 20 mcg; C 500 mg; bioflavonoids 50 mg.
    Increase high-fiber foods in diet.

25. If you get recurrent stomach or intestinal upsets and no physical cause can be found:
    Increase Vitamin B_1 10 mg; B_2 10 mg; B_5 20 mg; folic acid 100 mcg; PABA 50 mg; C 250 mg; bioflavonoids 25 mg.

26. If you get recurrent colds, flus:
    Increase Vitamin A 1,000 IU; B_3 50 mg; B_5 20 mg; B_6 10 mg; B_{12} 10 mcg; folic acid 50 mcg; choline 200 mg; C 1,000 mg; bioflavonoids 100 mg; calcium 200 mg; magnesium 100 mg; phosphorus 50 mg; zinc 10 mg.

27. If you get recurrent joint, back, neck aches and pains, especially on waking in the morning, and no physical cause can be found:
    Increase Vitamin A 1,000 IU; B_3 100 mg; B_5 30 mg; B_6 10 mg; calcium 200 mg; magnesium 100 mg; phosphorus 50 mg; zinc 10 mg; manganese 5 mg; molybdenum 50 mcg.

Avoid eating potatoes, tomatoes, red and green peppers, eggplant, paprika and chocolate, to avoid solanine.

28. If you get cramps or muscle twitches at night or "restless legs" or "go-to-sleep" extremities:
    Increase Vitamin B_1 20 mg; B_2 40 mg; E 200 IU; zinc 10 mg.
    Avoid caffeine intake—coffee, tea, colas, cocoa, chocolate.

29. If you get cold hands or feet or feel the cold more than most people:
    Increase Vitamin B_1 10 mg; B_2 10 mg; B_3 25 mg; B_5 25 mg; B_6 5 mg; B_{12} 10 mcg; folic acid 50 mcg; biotin 100 mcg; C 500 mg; bioflavonoids 50 mg; iodine 50 mg.
    Avoid eating *raw* vegetables of the genus *Brassica*—cabbage, turnips, kale, watercress.

30. Exercise
    - ☐ If you do heavy exercise for more than thirty minutes three times a week or more:
      Increase Vitamin B_1 50 mg; B_2 10 mg; B_3 50 mg; B_5 50 mg; B_6 5 mg; B_{12} 50 mcg; folic acid 100 mcg; biotin 500 mcg; C 1,000 mg; bioflavonoids 100 mg; E 200 IU; calcium 200 mg; magnesium 100 mg; potassium 50 mg; iron 5 mg.
    - ☐ If you feel you should exercise but can't face it no matter how hard you try—lie down for thirty minutes and the feeling should go away. Then read Chapters 4 and 5 again.

31. If you get sore or tender muscles for no apparent reason:
    Increase Vitamin B_1 30 mg; B_6 20 mg; biotin 200 mcg; D 200 IU.

32. If you are female:
    Increase Vitamin B_6 10 mg; folic acid 200 mcg; calcium 100 mg; magnesium 100 mg; iron 10 mg.

33. If you get bad menstrual cramps or premenstrual tension, then for three days before your period and all during your period:
    Increase Vitamin B_6 50 mg; E 100 IU; calcium 250 mg; magnesium 250 mg; iron 10 mg; zinc 20 mg.

34. Do you use a contraceptive pill?
    No: Gold Star
    Yes: Increase Vitamin B_1 30 mg; B_2 30 mg; B_6 10 mg; B_{12} 30 mcg; folic acid 100 mcg; C 500 mg; bioflavonoids 50 mg; E 100 IU; zinc 5 mg; chromium 25 mcg.

Add up all your increases carefully. Check additions, making sure not to confuse micrograms (mcg) with milligrams (mg). Now you have a basic formula. Before using it, modify it carefully in accord with the directions in Chapter 7. This will improve your nutrition considerably. Remember, the formula consists purely of nutrients. Unlike drugs, these work in conjunction with your body. Therefore, you should not get *any* unpleasant effects from taking them. If you do, stop taking them immediately. Recheck your formula and your source of vitamins and minerals to see that they conform to instructions given in this chapter and Chapter 7. If you wish, you can use the basic formula for three months. To refine it further then or now, press on with the next section.

The Refined Formula

Some of the questions in this section can be answered only by obtaining the information from a blood test and hair or tissue analysis.

1. If you are over forty and have noticed a decline in your memory:

   Increase Vitamin B_1 25 mg; folic acid 100 mcg; choline 500 mg; calcium 200 mg; manganese 5 mg.
   Add lecithin 1,000 mg.

2. If you get recurrent ringing or buzzing in your ears but *do not* take aspirin daily:

   Increase magnesium 100 mg; potassium 30 mg; manganese 10 mg.

3. If you get recurrent heart palpitations and no physical cause can be found:

   Increase Vitamin A 1,000 IU; C 500 mg; bioflavonoids 50 mg; D 100 IU; magnesium 100 mg; phosphorus 100 mg; iron 10 mg; manganese 5 mg.

4. If you often find it hard to get your breath or have shortness of breath or a "tight" chest and no physical cause can be found:

   Increase Vitamin B_{12} 20 mcg; folic acid 50 mcg; C 500 mg; bioflavonoids 50 mg; calcium 100 mg; zinc 5 mg.

5. If your cholesterol level is above 200 mg/dl:

   Increase Vitamin B_3 100 mg (niacin form only); choline 500 mg; inositol 500 mg; C 1,000 mg; bioflavonoids 100 mg.
   Add linoleic acid 400 mg; lecithin 1,000 mg; pectin 500 mg.
   Eat garlic and onions freely. Read Chapter 9.

6. If your triglycerides level is above 300 mg/dl:
   Increase inositol 500 mg.
   Increase high-fiber foods in your diet, e.g., whole grains, raw vegetables, brown rice.

7. Blood pressure (mm Hg)
   - ☐ 90–120/60–80: Gold Star
   - ☐ 121–125/75–80: O.K.
   - ☐ 126–139/75–89:
     Increase Vitamin B_5 50 mg; inositol 500 mg; C 500 mg; bioflavonoids 50 mg; calcium 250 mg.
     Reduce salt and caffeine in diet. Avoid all salty foods (see chapters 2 and 9).
   - ☐ Above 139/89. See a physician competently trained in nutrition.

8. If you use aspirin or items containing aspirin more than twice per week:
   Increase Vitamin C 500 mg; bioflavonoids 50 mg.
   Never take aspirin and Vitamin C at the same time.

9. If you are forever taking antihistamines for all sorts of vague complaints such as travel sickness:
   Increase calcium 200 mg.

10. If you use "water pills" (diuretics):
    Increase potassium 50 mg.
    Eat fresh, raw fruit daily.

11. Skin and mouth conditions
    - ☐ If you tend to get greasy dandruff and flaky skin on the forehead and around the nose and mouth, and pale cracked lips and corners of the mouth, look at your tongue. If it has a cherry-red tip:
      Increase Vitamin B_6 25 mg.

☐ If the mouth itself is also pale and tender to hot or cold liquids:
Increase Vitamin B_{12} 40 mcg.

☐ If you tend to get a sore mouth combined with a beef-red tongue and mouth plus stomach disturbances:
Increase Vitamin B_2 30 mg; B_3 50 mg; B_6 10 mg; folic acid 50 mcg.

☐ If you tend to get cracked lips and corners of the mouth with small red scaly patches on ears or eyelids and your eyes are very sensitive to bright light:
Increase Vitamin B_1 50 mg; B_2 50 mg; folic acid 100 mcg.

☐ If you tend to get recurrent grayish dry, scaly skin flakes on your face:
Increase biotin 500 mcg.

☐ If you tend to get canker sores in your mouth or herpes simplex (cold sores) on your lips:
Increase Vitamin B_3 50 mg.
Add lysine 250 mg.

☐ If you have an active herpes infection:
Increase lysine to 500 mg and see Appendix 2.

12. Eye Conditions

☐ If you get recurrent inflamed eyes or burning or a sandy feeling under the eyelids and no physical cause can be found:
Increase Vitamin A 1,000 IU; B_2 50 mg.

☐ If you have more difficulty seeing in darkness than most people:
Increase Vitamin A 1,000 IU; zinc 10 mg.

13. If you have a hand or head tremor and no physical cause can be found:
Increase choline 500 mg; magnesium 100 mg; zinc 10 mg.
Add lecithin 1,000 mg.

14. If your hair is graying prematurely and you have recurrent sensations of burning in your feet coupled with undue fatigue:

    Increase Vitamin B_5 50 mg; folic acid 50 mcg; PABA 50 mg.

15. If you get recurrent diarrhea but no physical cause can be found:

    Increase Vitamin B_3 100 mg.
    Add linoleic acid 400 mg.
    Avoid coffee.

16. If you get muscle weakness despite exercise and no physical cause can be found:

    Increase potassium 50 mg.

17. Hair and tissue conditions

☐ If you have had a hair or tissue test done and it shows an elevated level of cadmium:

    Increase Vitamin C 500 mg; bioflavonoids 50 mg; calcium 200 mg; iron 20 mg; zinc 10 mg; selenium 50 mcg.

☐ If you have had a hair or tissue test done and it shows an elevated level of mercury:

    Increase Vitamin C 500 mg; bioflavonoids 50 mg; zinc 20 mg; selenium 50 mcg.
    Avoid sources of mercury pollution, described in Chapter 3.

☐ If you have had a hair or tissue test done and it shows an elevated level of lead:

    Increase Vitamin C 500 mg; bioflavonoids 50 mg; E 200 IU; calcium 200 mg; phosphorus 100 mg; iron 15 mg; zinc 15 mg.
    Avoid sources of lead pollution, described in Chapter 3.

☐ If you have had a hair or tissue test done and it shows an elevated level of aluminum:

Increase Vitamin C 500 mg; bioflavonoids 50 mg; zinc 10 mg.

Avoid sources of aluminum pollution, described in Chapter 3.

☐ If you have had a hair or tissue test done and it shows an elevated level of arsenic:

Increase Vitamin C 500 mg; bioflavonoids 50 mg; selenium 60 mcg; iodine 100 mcg.

☐ If you have had a hair or tissue test done and it shows an elevated level of copper:

Increase zinc 20 mg; manganese 20 mg; molybdenum 50 mcg; selenium 50 mcg.

18. Hold your left hand out flat. Now bend the middle and top joints of your fingers, but not the knuckle joint. You should be able to touch the top of your palm with the bent fingertips without any stiffness or pain. Now do the other hand. If one or both hands have pain or stiffness in this movement:

Increase Vitamin B_3 50 mg; B_5 25 mg; B_6 15 mg.

☐ If you cannot touch the palms with the bent fingertips:

Increase Vitamin B_3 100 mg; B_5 50 mg; B_6 30 mg.

Reduce intake of potatoes, tomatoes, green and red peppers, eggplant, paprika and chocolate.

19. If you get recurrent headaches and no physical cause can be found:

Increase Vitamin B_2 50 mg; B_3 (niacin form) 50 mg; B_3 (niacinamide form) 100 mg.

20. If you are over sixty and have a lot of "age spots" on your skin (brown fatty pigment) coupled with *two* or more of: loss of balance, blurred vision, memory deficit, ringing or buzzing in ears, enlarged middle joints on your fingers (Heberden's nodes), but no physical causes can be found:

Increase Vitamin B_1 20 mg; B_3 100 mg; B_5 50 mg; B_6 10 mg; B_{12} 50 mcg; folic acid 50 mcg; C 1,000 mg; bioflavonoids 100 mg; E 200 IU; calcium 500 mg; magnesium 350 mg; zinc 25 mg; molybdenum 50 mcg; selenium 50 mcg; chromium 50 mcg.
Add a digestive enzyme tablet giving at least 2,000 units of lipase activity.

21. If you suspect you are a little allergic to any particular food, measure your pulse while sitting *before* you eat it. Then measure your pulse in the same position thirty to sixty minutes after eating it and without any intervening physical activity such as walking about. If it is *more than* ten beats higher than before the meal, avoid that food.

So now you have it, the personal formula. If you answered and totaled accurately, it should be immensely beneficial. Chapter 7 tells you what kinds of vitamins and minerals you need to make it up. Check each one carefully, because there are some restrictions on what forms and amounts are beneficial. Always take the formula immediately *after* a main meal, with a *large* glass of water, juice or milk. Better, divide it equally in two and take one half after breakfast and the other half after dinner. Never take it without food and drink.

An excellent way to ensure that you take the supplement regularly is to buy 2″ x 2″ sealable polythene packets and pack thirty days of individual supplements from the various bottles. A day's packet will slip into purse or pocket, ready to go anywhere. For trips away, a week's packets take up almost no room in a travel bag. Combined with good eating habits, these individually designed supplements are the best health insurance money can buy.

CHAPTER 7

THE VITAMINS AND MINERALS

In 1747, when naval physician Dr. James Lind first proposed that scurvy could be cured with oranges, limes and green vegetables, he was ostracized by his colleagues for tainting the noble profession of medicine with worthless folklore. "Cure a disease with a vegetable—preposterous." It took another 48 years of evidence before the navy made limes a daily ration for British sailors. Hence the name "Limey." The essential ingredient in limes, Vitamin C, was not isolated for another 133 years, in 1928, by Albert Szent-Gyorgyi.

At one time beriberi also was thought to be an infectious disease. Solemn scientific papers attested that the microbe had been identified. When Japanese researcher Kanehiro Takaki published evidence in the British medical journal *Lancet* in 1877 that diet could prevent beriberi, he was ridiculed. Thirty-five years of evidence later, biochemist Casimir Funk isolated a substance in rice hulls that stops beriberi, the vitamin we now call thiamine.

This sad history continues today: pompous ridicule and enormous lag before the acceptance of nutritional discoveries. Dr. Roger Williams isolated pantothenic acid (B_5) in 1938. It has since been discovered that a B_5 deficiency in animals causes multiple symptoms leading to organ failure and sudden death.[1] Similar deficiency symptoms have been experimentally induced in human subjects.[2] The National Academy of Sciences suggests

4–7 mg of Vitamin B_5 a day as an *average* allowance.[3] Studies of some American diets show that they contain even less than this small amount.[4] Yet although pantothenic acid is nontoxic up to at least *ten grams* a day,[5] after forty-five years it is still waiting to get on the RDA table.[6]

You don't have to wait. Having done your initial formula, now read what forms of the nutrients you should take to get the greatest benefits. Although each one is discussed separately, remember always that it is the multiple interactions of nutrients that is the basis of their biological activity. Now, with the aid of computers, we know that old practices, such as giving supplements of iron alone during pregnancy, are counterproductive. Never take single-nutrient supplements. By designing your own complete supplement, based on your body, your life stage, your deficits, your habits, you are participating in the beginning of a development in nutrition science aimed at controlling the basis of life itself.

"Natural" or Synthetic Nutrients?

Most claims that vitamins are "natural" are untrue. All vitamins today are predominantly synthetic. For example, Vitamin C labeled "with" rose hips or acerola simply means that 99 percent or more of synthetic Vitamin C has been blended with a sprinkling of rose-hip or acerola powder. You can't make C tablets any other way. Rose-hip powder contains only 25–50 mg of C per 100 grams (3½ oz). One 1,000-mg C tablet made entirely of rose hips would weigh 9 lbs and be the size of a football. I can't think how you would eat it.

Acerola extract, the most potent natural source, is about 20 percent Vitamin C. So, a pound of pure acerola would make eighty whopping, 1,000-mg tablets, far too big to swallow. But the worst problem is the enormous cost of acerola. Manufacturers pay more than thirty dollars a pound for it. You would pay sixty dollars at least for a finished product. If your supplement has 5,000 mg C in it, then that vitamin alone in the form of acerola would cost you $1,380 a year.

"Natural" multivitamins are also predominantly synthetic. Often they appear to claim liver or natural yeast as the source. The fine print usually says "with" rather than "made from." Take niacin, for example, the most concentrated of the B vitamins in yeast. One hundred grams (3½ oz) of good brewers' or torula yeast contains about 40 mg of niacin.[7] A multivitamin pill containing 200 mg of natural yeast niacin would weigh more than a pound. A jar of one hundred such pills would be the size of a small refrigerator. "Natural" vitamins sold today are not in any way a superior product to reputable synthetic vitamins. They are, however, up to three times the price. Seems an awful lot to charge for a few cunning words and a pretty label.

Another common claim is that we should use natural vitamins because they contain as-yet-unknown nutritional factors. Undoubtedly, they do. But the tiny sprinkling of the natural substances in the mass of synthetic pills *called* natural is negligible. In any case, unknown nutrients are best caught by eating a wide range of fresh, raw foods, not by relying on them to survive the refining processes that go into making a pill. There is no way of testing to see if they do survive, because we don't know what they are. As Marshall McLuhan taught us, the unknown-nutrient argument is just another way of selling the sound of sizzle for more than the sausage.

Vitamin A (Retinol), Provitamin A (Carotenoids)

Vitamin A maintains the skin and mucous membranes and a substance called visual purple in the eye which is required for night vision. Vitamin A is an oil-soluble nutrient that can build up in the body. For adults, beyond 85,000 IU a day of Vitamin A can quickly become toxic. For children, beyond 15,000 IU of Vitamin A can be toxic. Symptoms of Vitamin A toxicity include dizziness, severe headache, nausea and vomiting.[8] Vitamin A occurs in the form of retinol (named after the retina of the eye) or carotenoids (named after carrots, the best source), both with different levels of activity in the body. Because of this, the old method of measuring the quantity, the International Unit (IU), is not strictly accurate. The new measure is retinol equivalents (RE), 1 RE = 3.33 IU retinol or 10 IU beta carotene. So, a supplement of, say, 10,000 IU retinol plus 10,000 IU carotenoids equals 4,000 RE Vitamin A.

The best supplemental form is a half-and-half mixture of retinol and carotenoids. For acne sufferers, the cis retinoic acid form is most effective. The best natural form, though not the most concentrated, is carrots. One good carrot can contain 20,000 IU Vitamin A activity. Wise parents who feed their children lots of raw carrots instead of cookies sometimes get the fright of a child whose forehead, nose, chin and palms turn yellow as the carotenoid pigment exudes from sweat glands. Where the sweat glands are concentrated, it leaves a yellow stain. Harmless, but a sign to switch to fruit and nuts for a week or two.

Vitamin B_1 (Thiamine)

Vitamin B_1 maintains normal carbohydrate metabolism and nervous-system function. It has no known toxicity,[9] but amounts over 1,000 mg may produce a mild diuretic effect (increases urination). Water-soluble like all the B vitamins, thiamine is readily lost from the body and must be replaced daily. No supplemental form is better than another. The best natural source of Vitamin B_1 is whole grains. Thiamine colors the urine bright yellow. This effect is harmless.

Vitamin B_2 (Riboflavin)

Vitamin B_2 is essential to cell maintenance and energy metabolism. It is required for all cell repair after injury. It has no known toxicity.[10] Any supplemental form will suffice. The best natural sources of Vitamin B_2 are milk and eggs. Riboflavin harmlessly yellows the urine.

Vitamin B_3 (Niacin, Niacinamide, Nicotinic Acid)

Vitamin B_3 is a component of two important coenzymes (helpers) in the body. It is involved in a wide variety of bodily processes and is present in every one of your sixty trillion cells. B_3 has very low toxicity, even at amounts of 3,000 mg.[11] It sometimes has side effects, however, in people with peptic ulcers and in diabetics. Individuals with these disorders should see a physician competent in nutrition before using niacin. The niacin and nicotinic-acid forms may cause a skin flush and sometimes an itch, even at 25 mg, in some people. This effect seems harmless and usually disappears in an hour. Niacinamide has no flushing effect and is therefore preferred by many. Clearly, this difference between the forms indicates different physiological effects. Niacinamide, for example, does not improve the metabolism of fats in the blood. Niacin does. Your supplement should contain niacin and niacinamide equally. If the flush bothers you, reduce the proportion of niacin or use a slow-release form. The best natural sources of Vitamin B_3 are peanuts and poultry.

Vitamin B_5 (Pantothenic Acid)

Vitamin B_5 is essential for energy metabolism and for the formation of acetylcholine, the substance involved in memory that was discussed in Chapter 4. It has no known toxicity up to ten grams a day. Higher doses may cause occasional diarrhea or water retention.[12] Any supplemental form is as good as another. The best natural sources of Vitamin B_5 are poultry, fish and whole grains. Pantothenic acid is concentrated in the human brain and may have important functions there in addition to its role with acetylcholine. Eating lots of foods containing pantothenic acid will not help your brain function, however, as it works only in combination with many other nutrients.

Vitamin B_6 (Pyridoxine, Pyridoxol, Pyridoxamine)

Vitamin B_6 is essential as a coenzyme (helper) for many of the enzymes involved in protein, fat and sugar metabolism. It has low toxicity, but your supplement should not contain more than 300 mg per day, because it has not been thoroughly investigated above this level.[13] No supplemental form is better than another. The best natural sources of Vitamin B_6 are wheat germ, walnuts and fish.

Vitamin B_6 is a group of three naturally occurring chemicals called pyridines. Each has different physiological functions, but their significance for health is still unknown. Some reports indicate involvement in brain function. Large doses of B_6 may produce very vivid dreams and night restlessness.[14]

Vitamin B_{12} (Cobalamins)

Vitamin B_{12} is a group of substances containing the mineral cobalt (hence the name cobalamins). Cobalamins have important roles in protein and fatty acid metabolism and in the production of red blood cells. There is no known toxicity for this vitamin.[15] Any supplemental form is as good as another. Poor absorption is the major problem. There is no evidence that sublingual (under the tongue) dissolving tablets increase absorption, even though their manufacturers claim they contain the intrinsic factor necessary for B_{12} absorption. The best natural sources of vitamin B_{12} are liver, clams and oysters. Liver, however, may be a bad food for other reasons discussed in Chapter 12.

Folic Acid (Folacin)

Folic acid is a cofactor (helper substance) of the B complex. It is itself a complex family of substances which are essential to the formation of red blood cells. Unfortunately, if taken in amounts over 1 mg a day, folic acid may mask the signs of pernicious anemia, which often results from deficiency of Vitamin B_{12}. Extra folic acid may prevent diagnosis of this disease before irreversible damage has occurred. If you do not have pernicious anemia, folic acid has no known toxicity up to 5 mg a day. Beyond this level it has not been thoroughly assessed. Any supplemental form is as good as another. The best natural sources of folic acid are raw green vegetables and raw fruit.

Biotin

Biotin is essential to the metabolism of carbohydrates and fats. It has no known toxicity. Any supplemental form is as good as another. The best natural sources of biotin are soybeans and brown rice. Raw egg white contains a substance called avidin which prevents biotin from being absorbed by the body. Recent cases of biotin deficiency in infants[16] have renewed interest in this cofactor of the B vitamins. Despite commercial razzmatazz, biotin does not prevent falling hair. Only complete nutrient supplements prevent degeneration.

Choline

Choline is a cofactor of the B vitamins which is crucial to normal brain function and memory. It also participates in the metabolism of fat and cholesterol. It has no known toxicity. The best supplemental form is phosphatidyl choline. The best natural sources of choline are lecithin and eggs. Recent reports of memory improvement induced by choline indicate that eating large choline supplements provides only a small part of the nutrient formula necessary to maintain memory.[17]

Inositol

Inositol, another cofactor of the B complex, works with choline in the metabolism of fat and cholesterol. It has widespread but still obscure functions in the body. Your nerves contain fifty times the inositol level of the blood. Inositol is essential to proper conduction of nerve impulses. The level in nerves declines with age and so does your speed of reaction. Human semen contains more inositol than any other vitamin or mineral, but we don't really know why. It has no known toxicity. No supplemental form is better than another. The best natural sources of inositol are lecithin and wheat germ.

Para-amino-benzoic acid (PABA)

This cofactor of the B vitamins is important for normal skin and hair growth and color in animals, but its functions in humans remain obscure. Spread on the skin PABA is *the* most effective sunscreen agent, but what it does within the body has yet to be established. It has no known toxic effects. Any supplemental form is as good as another. The best natural sources of PABA are whole grains and wheat germ.

Vitamin C (Ascorbic Acid)

Like the B vitamins, ascorbic acid is water-soluble and easily lost from the body. It must be replaced daily for optimum health. It is widely involved in almost every bodily function. More than ten grams a day of Vitamin C can produce diarrhea in some people, owing to direct acitvity in the digestive tract and excretion through the bowels. It also has a mild diuretic effect. Aside from these effects it is nontoxic. People have now taken ten grams of Vitamin C daily for thirty years without any toxic effects,[18] and, indeed, with a great deal of benefit. The calcium ascorbate form of Vitamin C is better tolerated than the ascorbic acid form. Don't take the sodium ascorbate form. You get too much sodium in your food already. The best natural sources of Vitamin C are citrus fruits (oranges, grapefruit, lemons, limes, tomatoes).

Bioflavonoids

Bioflavonoids are a complex family of chemicals including substances called rutin and hesperidin. They have numerous but still undefined activities in the body, including protective effects on Vitamin C stores and on the strength of capillaries. They are widely distributed in fresh raw fruits and vegetables and have no known toxicity. The best supplemental form is mixed bioflavonoids included in a Vitamin C preparation.

Vitamin D (Calciferol)

This fat-soluble vitamin is now known to have hormone effects also. That is, it has specific messenger and regulatory functions as well as its general effects as a vitamin. Its main function in the body is regulating calcium and phosphate metabolism. It is formed on human skin by the ultraviolet light in sunlight reacting with cholesterol (yes, cholesterol) in the skin. Above 30,000 IU in adults and 2,000 IU in children, Vitamin D is toxic.[19] Some rare people show signs of poisoning at 5,000 IU. Vitamin D is now measured as micrograms of cholecalciferol activity: 10 mcg = 400 IU. There are two common supplemental forms of Vitamin D, ergocalciferol (D_2) and cholecalciferol (D_3). Each is equally good. It is sold only in conjunction with Vitamin A or in a multipreparation. The best natural source is sunlight. The vitamin D added to milk is a fair source.

Vitamin E (Tocopherol)

This fat-soluble vitamin is still not recognized as essential by many countries.[20] It has widespread actions in the body and is crucial to normal procreation. It has no known toxicity, but may raise high blood pressure in some cases, in amounts above 1,200 IU. Vitamin E may also affect some other medical conditions, namely diabetes and thyroid dysfunctions. So, if you have any of these, get your physician's advice before using Vitamin E as a supplement.

In nature Vitamin E occurs as a family of fat-soluble substances called tocopherols found mainly in wheat germ, vegetable oils, leafy green vegetables and whole grains. The main ones are alpha-, beta-, delta- and gamma-tocopherol. All have different activity levels. That is why Vitamin E is measured in international units of activity rather than in milligrams. The United States has just adopted a new measure in milligram equivalents of alpha-tocopherol activity (TE): 1 mg d-alpha-tocopherol = 1 alpha TE.

The "d" in d-alpha-tocopherol is important. It designates the dextro form of alpha-tocopherol that occurs in nature. This is the one case where a natural vitamin is better than the synthetic. Synthetic E contains both dextro-alpha-tocopherol and a levo-alpha-tocopherol that is not usable by the body. And the proportion of each form is uncertain in synthetic preparations. So buy only Vitamin E which states it is d-alpha-tocopherol (*not* dl-alpha-tocopherol). If the label doesn't say, you can bet it is the dl-alpha-tocopherol, because that is a lot cheaper to produce. And buy it fresh. Vitamin E starts to oxidize in the capsules within a few months of manufacture. Taking old E capsules is eating the very toxins that you take Vitamin E to protect you from.

Minerals

"Chelated" is a good selling word for mineral supplements. It means that the mineral has been combined with another substance, usually with an amino acid, to increase its bioavailability. There is some evidence that the absorption of *some* chelated minerals is improved. The process may be facilitated further if the supplement is "hydrolyzed," meaning it dissolves more easily in water. Bioavailability, however, as we have seen, depends heavily on the type and quantity of foods taken with the supplements. Do not be too concerned if your mineral supplement is not chelated, and don't reduce the quantity just because it is. All the mineral quantities referred to in this book are "elemental," that is, are amounts that would be bioavailable if absorption were perfect. Buy only those that state the elemental amount made available by the supplement. Now let's look at the minerals individually.

Calcium

More than 95 percent of your calcium is in your bones and teeth, but it also has widespread functions in the cardiovascular system and the nervous system. As soon as you stop using the skeleton, that is, moving it against gravity, bones lose calcium fast. One of the big problems of long, weightless spaceflight is that astronauts may return to earth with bones too weak to hold up their bodies. Maintaining the calcium in bone structure is one of the major reasons you should walk at least thirty minutes a day. You can't do it just by eating calcium. The essential interaction of skeletal mineralization and exercise is a big reason why it doesn't work to simply give old people calcium supplements to strengthen their fragile bones.

Like all minerals, calcium should never be taken alone, as it can have a variety of toxic effects. With a complete supplement it is nontoxic up to 15,000 mg a day of calcium gluconate.[21] Prolonged use, however, can result in calcium overload (hypercalcemia). A good form of calcium is dolomite, which also provides magnesium in the correct ratio. But the body will take its calcium in almost any form. Milk and cheese are good natural sources of calcium. Bone meal is not recommended because of the high lead content of animal bones today. Don't use calcium chloride or calcium lactate either. You don't need the chloride or the lactate, and both forms are inferior in calcium compared to calcium gluconate.

Magnesium

Magnesium is present everywhere in the body. It is involved in everything from protein synthesis and energy production to nervous function and muscle contraction. It can be toxic in amounts over ten grams of magnesium sulphate and smaller amounts in other forms,[22] especially if taken over a long period. Much of our food is deficient in this mineral. It is lost in the refining of grains and because the numerous chemicals used in food processing chelate it out of foods. If you have "hard" drinking water, it is protecting your heart and bones by providing magnesium and calcium. Dolomite is an excellent source of magnesium. Some natural sources are lemons, grapefruit and apples.

Phosphorus

Phosphorus is in every cell of the body, amounting to about two pounds in an average-sized person, mostly resident in the bones. There it works in multiple interactions with calcium. American diets, especially with high meat intake, are too high in phosphorus. So we tend to get calcium-depleted, one very good reason to avoid meat. Dolomite is a good source of phosphorus, as is yeast, but any phosphorus supplement will suffice. Despite possible excesses in the diet, phosphorus should be included in your supplement for completeness and balance. Good natural sources of phosphorus are fish and poultry.

Potassium

Your half-pound of potassium is so busy throughout your body that to cite just one of its functions, such as nerve conduction, is to do it injustice. Potassium deficiency is common in America because of the overuse of antibiotics and diuretics, both of which dispose of bodily potassium. Amounts up to 600 mg of potassium gluconate are nontoxic. Any supplemental form will suffice, but don't ever take a potassium supplement alone. It will burn hell out of your stomach and intestines. In a multimineral pill, right after food and drink and with the rest of your supplement, potassium is fine. Natural sources of potassium are leafy green vegetables, citrus fruits and bananas.

Iron

We have already covered iron in other chapters. One of its major functions is to make hemoglobin. Iron is lost whenever you lose blood. Iron stores are hard to replace too, because of iron's poor bioavailability. Malabsorption is an ever-increasing problem today, because our lead and cadmium pollution further reduce the availability of iron in food. Partly because of menstruation, women have a greater need for iron supplements than men. Any supplemental form is as good as another. Prolonged supplementation *in men* of more than 50 mg/day can lead to toxicity.[23] Most foods contain iron. Iron from meats, called heme iron, is better absorbed than the nonheme iron in vegetables.

Copper

This essential mineral has widespread body functions, including helping to convert iron to hemoglobin and promoting utilization of Vitamin C. Copper is present in excess in most American diets, largely from contamination of water passing through copper pipes. A little is included in your formula for completeness only; you don't need to take additional copper supplements.

Zinc

Zinc is essential for cell growth, protein synthesis and the utilization of Vitamin A. Unlike copper, zinc is very likely to be deficient in American diets. We have to supplement our livestock feed with this mineral to maintain good growth and health, because the grains themselves are deficient in zinc. In our own food, we stupidly remove even the deficient amount of zinc from the grains during processing and *don't add any back.* So we do need zinc supplements. Zinc will upset your stomach if you take it alone. You should not have more than 200 mg in your supplement. It is difficult to take too much zinc into the body, however, because, be warned, excesses eaten will be rapidly and uncomfortably excreted from both ends. Zinc sulphate is a good supplemental form. Natural sources of zinc are oysters, eggs and whole wheat.

Manganese

This essential metal is necessary throughout the body, from protein metabolism to glandular secretions to brain function.

Excess manganese interferes with iron absorption, but the mineral itself is of low toxicity. Nevertheless, you should not have more than 40 mg of manganese in your supplement. Any supplemental form is as good as another. Natural sources are tea, leafy green vegetables and whole grains, especially rice bran, wheat bran and oat bran. But American soils are deficient in manganese owing to overuse. So vegetables and grains vary widely in manganese content.

Molybdenum

This essential metal has diverse functions, including participation in three essential enzyme systems in the body. It is present in many foods and unlikely to be deficient, except in some conditions of mineral imbalance. Any supplemental form suffices, though few available supplements contain it. Your supplement should not contain more than 200 mcg.

Chromium

This metal is essential to sugar metabolism in the body. Body levels of chromium decline progressively with age in America, though not in some other countries. Chromium deficiency is now a suspected factor in our "epidemics" of glucose intolerance and adult-onset diabetes. Very recent evidence indicates that supplementing *normal* healthy Americans with chromium improves glucose tolerance.[24]

Chromium provides an excellent example of the rapidly changing face of nutrition science. In 1968 chromium rated only two sentences in the RDA handbook, which stated that studies on chromium "are suggestive of a possible role in human nutrition."[25] By 1980 chromium rated two pages of studies, and the RDA committee considered the mineral essential. It stated that "50–200 mcg a day is tentatively recommended for adults."[26]

Chromium still has not made the RDA table though, but it might by 1990. Your supplement should contain chromium in what is called the trivalent form, organically bound, often sold as "glucose tolerance factor" (GTF). Natural sources of chromium are shellfish, whole wheat bread and mushrooms.

Selenium

Selenium is another element that was considered only a "maybe" in human nutrition before 1970.[27] Now, we know it is crucial to enzymes that protect human cells against damage by free oxygen particles, and to normal heart function. Selenium is *very* toxic, however. Your daily supplement should not contain more than 300 mcg. People breathing the fumes of Xerox machines all day (which contain selenium) may easily overdose.[28] For many of us, selenium deficiency is more likely, owing to widespread selenium deficiencies in American soils. Supplements should contain organically bound selenium, usually obtained from brewers' yeast. Inorganic forms such as sodium selenite or selenium dioxide should not be used. They are more toxic and less bioavailable. A very good natural source of selenium is wheat germ.

Iodine

Best known for its essential role in thyroid function, iodine is a strange element. Excesses of iodine *damage* the thyroid. An iodate form of iodine was formerly used widely as a dough conditioner in breadmaking, and excesses (over 1,000 mcg) could occur from eating as little as six slices of bread. Up to 1,000 mcg of iodates is nontoxic.[29] Now, use of iodates is declining and many people restrict their (iodized) salt intake, so deficiency is likely. Any supplemental form of iodine will suffice. All seafoods are good natural sources.

Sodium, Chlorine

Both these minerals have multiple essential functions in the human body, and we need them daily in large amounts. Unfortunately, our diets are so loaded with hidden salt (sodium chloride) that we get too much of both. In addition, we have chlorine in the water supply. Anyone taking extra sodium or chlorine, except on medical advice for rare conditions, is damaging his or her health. Taking salt tablets for exhaustion or excessive sweating, for example, is a Victorian misinterpretation of science that should have died out in the last century, along with bloodletting.

Sulfur

This essential mineral with myriad functions in the body is no longer available as an over-the-counter food supplement. Yet it is required in large amounts, about 1,000 mg a day. Diets with 6 oz or more of complete protein, found in meat, fish and dairy products, provide ample sulfur in the amino acids methionine, cysteine, cystine and taurine. Eggs are a particularly good source of sulfur. Onions and garlic are good sources for vegetarians.

Fluorine

Fluorine is essential for maintenance of the bones and teeth. Calcium fluoride of 0.7 to 1.2 parts per million is now added to most water supplies. People who drink lots of tea, like the British, get ample fluorine already, up to 3 mg a day. Sea salt contains appreciable amounts too. Although fluorine protects teeth from the dental caries associated with our high-sugar diets, too much fluorine *causes* pitting and brown mottling of growing teeth. In areas of America with fluorine in the soil or water above four parts per million, many people have permanent fluorine "camouflage" on their smile. More important, the excess damages their bones also, and there is no effective treatment once that has happened.[30] Don't take fluorine supplements except on medical advice.

Vanadium, Nickel, Cobalt, Silicon

The essential minerals vanadium, nickel, cobalt and silicon are not available to the public in good supplemental forms in America, so it is pointless to recommend any. You have to get them from your diet. Vanadium is involved in cholesterol metabolism. It is widely available in unprocessed foods, especially *cold-pressed* soybean and olive oils, dill pickles and the humble radish.

Nickel is widely distributed in human functioning, and nickel deficiencies have been shown in several species of animal. But the precise functions of this mineral remain unknown. Nickel is abundantly available in unprocessed grains, but is lost in processing. It is relatively nontoxic by itself, but mixed with carbon monoxide it forms the carcinogen nickel carbonyl, which is responsible for the high rate of lung cancer among employees of nickel refineries. Smokers get nickel carbonyl as a nasty little extra from cigarette smoke.[31]

Cobalt is an integral component of Vitamin B_{12} and we can get all our cobalt requirement from this vitamin. Inorganic forms of cobalt cannot be utilized by humans and other one-stomach (monogastric) animals. Leafy green vegetables, liver and kidneys are the best dietary sources of cobalt, although the meats today contain chemical residues which do not recommend their use.

Silicon is essential for growth and skeletal maintenance in various animals. Daily requirements for human beings are unknown, but are probably fairly large. Some human adult diets contain over 1,000 mg of silicon a day without apparent problems.[32] Your silicon requirements are best obtained from unprocessed vegetables.

Other Essential Substances

Your formula may have come out containing lysine, one of the essential amino acids. It combines with Vitamin B_6 and an enzyme called lysyl oxidase to make elastin, an essential component of all your connective tissues. Certain viruses, including herpes (both the facial and genital types) and some other canker-sore viruses, are inhibited in the presence of lysine, and grow fast in the presence of arginine, another amino acid. Increasing dietary lysine with supplements while avoiding arginine-rich foods such as corn, rice, *canned* peas and beans, chocolate and nuts has successfully stopped herpes in careful clinical trials.[33] A full list of lysine-rich foods to use in curbing herpes is given in Appendix 2. It makes sense to use this harmless nutrient to avoid an annoying condition now epidemic in America. With anything but mild herpes, however, see a physician competently trained in nutrition immediately. Any form of lysine supplement will suffice.

Another possible component of your formula is linoleic acid. Linoleic acid and arachidonic acid are the two essential fatty acids that the body cannot make. It can however, make arachidonic acid from linoleic acid. Numerous people are deficient in these essential fatty acids. The best source of linoleic acid is an oil extracted from the evening primrose plant. It is nontoxic up to 5,000 mg.

Some formulas may contain pectin, a carbohydrate found in many fruits. It is not an essential nutrient, but is included because it affects the metabolism of fats and acts to lower cholesterol.[34] It is nontoxic. The best natural sources of pectin are grapefruit, oranges and apples.

You may also have lecithin in your formula. This phospholipid is made constantly by the body but is still low under some conditions. Supplements are beneficial in metabolism of the excess fats common in the American diet. Any form of lecithin will suffice. The usual natural source is soybeans. Lecithin is nontoxic up to 20,000 mg. Liquid lecithin makes an excellent cooking oil. It is very slippery stuff too. Pancakes and omelets cooked in lecithin never stick to the pan.

Finally, your formula may contain digestive enzymes for certain conditions that suggest a possible decline in pancreas function, and therefore digestive degeneration and malabsorption of nutrients. The pancreas, however, has a very large reserve capacity. Malabsorption does not start to occur until the output of digestive enzymes by the pancreas is reduced to only 10 percent.[35] So, despite the enzyme fad promoted by some health-food magazines, supplemental enzymes are rarely needed. When they are, most of the over-the-counter preparations are useless, because they don't have sufficient levels of lipase activity, the most important substance. Buy one only if its stated contents include at least 2,000 units of lipase activity per dose. Festal (Hoechst) and Cotazym (Organon) meet this criterion. Tablets work better than capsules, and enteric-coated pills are no good because they just don't dissolve quickly enough or in the right place to help digest the food.[36]

Other Substances in the Biochemical Equation

We investigate so many substances in our quest to prevent degeneration that our laboratory hello is, "What's the wonder drug today?" From ginseng to Gerovital we chase them down Hunza valleys, up Tibetan peaks and through the laboratories of billion-dollar conglomerates. I wish I could tell you that we've found the elixir. Without a commitment to science it would be tempting to make such a claim, with a hundred million souls eager to buy it.

Ginseng, for example, has been used for five thousand years

to avert aging. Most pills, capsules and teas you can buy in America contain negligible quantities of the active ingredients of ginseng. These are called saponins, powerful substances that have a multitude of biological actions, none of which is understood. A packet of the popular instant ginseng tea contains no saponins at all that we can detect, even with the most sensitive laboratory analyses. These instant ginseng teas are actually 99 percent plain old sugar. Any lift you get from them is from drinking flavored sugar water.

There are two ginsengs with known, long-acting stimulant effects, *Panax schinseng,* the original Chinese source, and *Panax quinquefolius,* the American variant. Few reputable studies have been done, but there is some evidence that the saponins in these plants may influence degeneration.[37] Two other plants cash in on this evidence: *Eleutherococcus senticosus,* called "Russian" or "Siberian" ginseng, and *Rumex hymenosepalus,* called "Wild Red" or "American Wild" ginseng. The first is a common Siberian weed. The second is the American weed red dock. There is no evidence that either has any beneficial activity in the human body. Red dock is not even a member of the ginseng family of plants (*Araliaceae*). Both are cheap, and are all you will be getting (mixed with a sprinkling of real ginseng) in any cheap product. They are quite useless.

We have traced the best of the real stuff to its guarded, pampered glory in state-run Korean farms and to almost-secret farms in America. Only the root or the concentrated extract have appreciable saponin activity. You will not get potent extract for less than sixty dollars an ounce. The best roots fetch enormous sums. Until there are reliable studies on dosage, form and effects, don't waste your money.

Another "elixir" is Gerovital H3, developed in Rumania by Dr. Anna Aslan.[38] It is now so popular that you can buy it without a prescription throughout Europe and Britain, and in Nevada, the only American state that has legalized its use. The active ingredient of the Aslan formula is a 2 percent solution of the local anesthetic drug procaine hydrochloride (Novocain) together with 0.3 percent potassium metabisulfite, 0.3 percent disodium phosphate and 0.3 percent benzoic acid as buffers and preservatives. The *maximum* single dose is 600 mg. I am stating the formula to show how simple a substance it is. Only the injectable forms have any proven value. The pill and capsule forms available recently are largely commercial humbug, because the procaine is slaughtered by the digestive process and doesn't get into the body at all.

Injected Gerovital has multiple effects, some stimulant, some suppressant. Its popularity with the aging celebrities who have eulogized its use probably stems from relief of depression. Clinical trials indicate that it has an antidepressant action, without side effects.[39] There is also *some* evidence that it relieves the pain of arthritis.[40] As yet, there is no reliable evidence that Gerovital has any effect in retarding degeneration or preventing disease. We have examined people who have used it for between five and thirty-four years. They claim considerable benefit. But we cannot find any indication that it has retarded aging.

The notion that a single drug like Novocain could prevent degeneration exemplifies the sort of obsolete thinking about human health this book seeks to expose. It is like Ponce de Leon searching vainly for the fountain of youth, when all along it was in his own bloodstream. At least sixty thousand different chemicals spell the biochemical equation of the human body. From a daily modicum of proteins, carbohydrates and fats, plus the vitamins and essential minerals, the body *makes* all the rest. What an awesome chemical factory, every chemical link interdependent in the chain of life. Yet we search constantly for other, artificial chemicals, drugs that have no place in the chain, to "improve" on a structure forged by three million years of evolution. We petty men, still incapable of using our intelligence to live in harmony with each other, would strut before nature, challenging her vast enterprise with our backyard chemistry.

Cooperation with nature is the only solution she will allow.

Drugs have no business in the healthy human body. Every needless drug you take, for an ache here, an itch there, damages you. In 1980 the Sixth World Nutrition Congress reported that even a single aspirin can make your intestines bleed *for a week!*[41] If you want a long and healthy life, leave drugs to the truly ill. They may benefit from them. You won't.

SECTION TWO

Four Big Killers and Lots of Little Ones

CHAPTER 8

THE BATTLE OF THE BULGE

THE PERENNIAL POPULARITY of health clubs and fat farms, slimming foods and steam baths, diets, pills and potions, shows how badly millions of us would like to be slimmer. Yet as a nation we are even fatter than we were twenty years ago. Now, nearly a third of all women and a sixth of all men are not just overweight but technically obese, that is, more than 25 percent above their ideal weights.[1] The men are gaining faster too. Compared with 1959, their weights are higher at all ages. While women now are heavier in their twenties, by their forties they are starting to hold their own in the battle of the bulge.[2]

Before we draw a straight correlation between weight and bodily degeneration, there is some good news. For many years the Metropolitan Life Insurance Company directed by the late Louis Dublin published charts suggesting imminent disaster from the smallest spare tire around your midriff—and charged premiums accordingly. There may still be such a chart on your doctor's wall. In 1980 superb analyses by a world expert on obesity, Dr. Ancel Keys, showed these charts to be wrong. Not only are the ideal weights about five to ten pounds too low, but up to twenty pounds of excess weight has no correlation with premature death. Obesity remains a serious threat to health, but a bit of extra padding is no mortal danger.[3] However, if you have gained a lot more than twenty pounds since college, don't despair. The following pages explode the expensive myths about overweight and give you the fat facts. Stay with them and you will have to buy a slimmer wardrobe.

What Obesity Does to You

Obesity is America's heaviest health burden. It predisposes you to heart disease, the atherosclerosis type of arteriosclerosis, hypertension, strokes, heart attacks, diabetes, bladder disease and cancer.[4] The very metabolism of fat cells destroys substances in the bloodstream that protect you from heart disease.[5] Fat increases the risk of disability or death in almost all diseases.[6] Obesity is the major form of malnutrition in America. It results from eating excess calories without nutriment, and is the overriding evidence for the degradation of our food supply.

The fatter a person becomes, the more his immune system becomes defective.[7] As we have seen, the results of defective immunity are susceptibility to infection and invasion of the body by toxins, both leading to rapid degeneration. For instance, in overweight people the chance of postoperative wound infections is increased by up to 700 percent,[8] making postoperative complications more serious, increasing time in the hospital and sometimes causing death.

You don't have to go to hospitals to see how overweight reduces resistance to illness. Giving the lie to the "healthy fat cheeks" image of childhood, in 1971 Dr. V. Tracey and his colleagues at Northampton General Hospital in Britain studied normal children from three months to two years old. They showed that fat babies get twice as many infections as slim ones.[9] One big reason breastfeeding breeds healthier babies is that it keeps them slimmer.[10]

In 1979 America's medical best gathered in force to consider dietary factors related to the nation's health. After reviewing volumes of evidence, they concluded that high cholesterol leads to arteriosclerosis. High saturated fat leads to arteriosclerosis. High salt leads to hypertension for many people. High carbohydrate leads to diabetes for some. But the "winner" in the disease stakes is plain old empty excess calories. Unequivocally, empty calories bring obesity, hypertension, diabetes and arteriosclerosis.[11] If you eat them, likely you will wear them, and all their attendant health problems.

Usual Responses to Overweight

Want to shed poundage? Stiffen the upper lip, join a health club, switch to no-cal sweeteners, take appetite suppressants, have psychotherapy, count calories meticulously, diet vigorously. So sing the litanies of the weight-loss marketplace. They must be unsuccessful, because we're getting fatter. Let's look at each in turn to find out why.

Health clubs are booming. Yet apart from lunch and rush hours, they are practically empty. A perusal of the records of one New York chain of clubs shows that most members appear, dressed for battle, *less than once a week.* One reason health clubs don't work is that many members just don't go. For them membership is a way of *avoiding* losing weight. Perhaps paying the fee confers a psychological satisfaction that something is being done.

What of the hardier souls that do attend? Surreptitious stopwatches held on people at New York health clubs show an average exercise time of *twelve minutes.* Spectating will not affect overweight, nor will lying on the floor breathing deeply. Yoga postures are beautiful, but they burn few calories. Propping up the juice bar *puts on* weight. Better than not going at all, but unlikely to shift an ounce.

Some health-club members go in for the vibrating gismos or surrender to vigorous massage to pound the fat away, or bake in the sauna to sweat it out. Our clinics use a sealed nylon sack full of wet sponges to show the uselessness of this approach. Massage it hard with vibrating rollers or hands, and you force water through the nylon. Put it in the sauna for an hour, and water evaporates through the nylon. In both cases, water goes and the sack loses weight. But pour more water in, and the newly thirsty sponges grab every drop. The weight is on again. The analogy is accurate. All you lose from pummel and sweat is water. And it is highly dangerous to your health to refuse to drink liquids to keep *that* (water-loss) weight off. So treat the gismos with contempt, realize the sauna is great for a chat, take massage for its sensual pleasures, but don't believe they will help you lose weight.

Artificial sweeteners don't help either. Both cyclamates and saccharin cause cancer in laboratory animals and are associated with increased incidence of bladder cancer in human patients. Cyclamates are banned though not yet abandoned. Saccharin was saved from an FDA ban in 1979, only because diabetics and the very obese claimed it as their lifeline. The new sweetener "aspartame" is no contender for a replacement, because it breaks down under heat and loses its sweetness. The main problem with artificial sweeteners, however, is not the risk of cancer, but the myth that they help to reduce weight. This notion seems logical in terms of calories and is well advertised, so it has become a popular belief. Yet in the last twenty years of soaring growth of saccharin sales, America has steadily gotten fatter. There is accumulating evidence, including some from my own clinics, that the calories saved by saccharin are more than replaced by extra eating, because the artificial sweetener fails to satisfy the mouth, throat and stomach mechanisms of appetite.

Cigarettes, amphetamines and the popular appetite suppressants all hold down the appetite, but only as long as you take the drugs. As soon as you stop, appetite rebounds above normal and you put on more weight than if you never used them. Over-the-counter appetite suppressants come in two main forms, chewables and swallowables. The chewables mostly contain benzocaine, a local anesthetic aimed at reducing the taste-bud response to food. Popular swallowables contain phenylpropanolamine (PPA). This drug acts partly as a stimulant, and partly to reduce the appetite response by affecting an area of the brain just behind your nose called the hypothalamus. Both drugs work short-term to *suppress* appetite. But after a few weeks the body works out that it has been fooled. Drug tolerance rises because the body starts to metabolize it and excrete it more efficiently. Rebound overeating follows, as the newly released appetite keeps you hovering round the fridge with unquenchable munchies.

A common response is to pop more PPA. Don't. Many recent studies show that PPA dangerously raises blood pressure.[12] As overweight people tend to be hypertensive already, this is doubly dangerous. In 1980, at the University of Melbourne in Australia, Dr. J. Horowitz and his colleagues tested a single 85-mg capsule of PPA (Trimolets) on thirty-seven healthy medical students. In twelve students there was a rapid rise in diastolic blood pressure of over 30 mm Hg. Three students required treatment for hypertensive crisis. More than half the students reported negative symptoms, including dizziness, palpitations and nausea.[13] Like many American physicians, these investigators concluded the drug should be banned from public sale. Not only is it useless for long-term weight control, it is also highly toxic.

Recently, there has been a rash of substances, usually derived from beans, which are supposed to inhibit the absorption of carbohydrates and, therefore, inhibit weight gain. *Don't use them.* True, they do inhibit some enzyme activity in the digestive tract. This action has been known for many years. But that only leaves the carbohydrate to putrefy farther down. Aside from the gas problem, the human colon was not designed to deal with continual masses of putrefying processed carbohydrate. Using a pill as an excuse to binge on junk food will not keep you slim or healthy.

In despair some of the overweight turn to psychotherapy. Since Freud, people have been blaming overweight on the unconscious. Unfortunately, slim people have the same amount of infantile trauma, stress, repressed desires, anxieties, fears and mental hobgoblins as fat ones. Both fat and slim alike binge their frustrations away. The slim stay so because internal physiological mechanisms stop their binging long before they get fat. There is not a single reliable study to show that neuroses accumulate poundage. Emotional problems of fatties are as much a result of wrong dieting as a cause of fat. Overweight people tend to diet. Most diets upset the body's physiological dynamics. After a week or two of starvation the body reacts by causing an irresistible urge to eat. We call this the *starvation failure complex.* Forget psychological explanations. Fat is a physical problem.

Throw Away Your Calorie Charts

Fat is not the difference between calories in, calories out. The body is far more cunning than that. To examine the effects of caloric restriction, we did a study at the University of Auckland with four men between ages twenty-four and forty and two women aged twenty-three and twenty-six, all with sedentary occupations. All four thought they could benefit by losing a few pounds. For six weeks they cut their usual lunch calories exactly in half, and maintained usual eating patterns for all other meals. They kept food diaries as a check. The reduction was between 200 and 450 calories a day. We were amazed to find that only two people lost any weight at all, and then only ¾ lb and 1½ lbs. In terms of missed calories, at 3,500 calories to the pound, they should have lost 2½ and 4½ lbs respectively. The others should have lost between 2¼ and 5½ lbs, but lost nothing at all.

Sorry, dieters, that's the fact. Removing calories from your food does not mean you will lose the equivalent in fat. The body has lots of defensive mechanisms to protect its fat stores. It's the same the other way around too. Try to force the body to put on weight and it is equally resistant. Many reports show it will dispose of extra calories by speeding up metabolism.[14]

Against such physiological dynamics, counting the calorie content of foods is a silly procedure. But it always was. It's worse than trying to estimate nutrient content. A "piece" of cherry pie, for example, can vary from 250 to 450 calories, depending on size, added sugar, type of pastry, type of cherries, and a dozen other ifs and buts.[15] Then too, you never know how many of the calories are bioavailable. Say you overdo your daily intake by just two hundred calories, the margin of error in a piece of pie. Theoretically, every week you would be storing an extra fourteen hundred calories, over a pound of fat every three weeks. In a year you would gain eighteen pounds. In ten years you would be a monster, 180 pounds obese. It just doesn't happen. Fortunately, the body is much better at counting calories than charts, and at taking steps to deal with them.

We Live on a FATPOINT

An unfortunate tiny few of us grow fat from glandular dysfunction or rare diseases. But the majority gain weight from overeating. Despite repeated dieting, they gradually lose the battle. To understand why, we need to remember the principles of biochemical individuality and physiological dynamics.

Because of biochemical individuality, people differ widely in their inherited *capacity* to accumulate fat through overeating. But the *amount* of fat gained is not preordained by the genes. This assumption is a common error of many old theories of fatness,[16] and even some variants of the recent "setpoint" theory.[17] Such theories assume individuals are destined to be comfortable only at certain levels of fat fixed by inheritance, and that their bodies will drive them mercilessly to that level (the "setpoint"). Now, we know that neither the number of fat cells nor their size is fixed.[18] What we inherit is different levels of tendencies to store fat. Whether we do or not depends on our lifestyle, not on any inborn urge to stuff.

From the principle of physiological dynamics, the body has no reference system for a fixed level of fat, only for a *usual* level. Form follows function for fat as well as muscle. When you get to adult weight and remain there for more than a year, the body develops all the enzyme systems, the new capillaries, the new peripheral nerves, the extra blood supply, the hormone levels, the muscles and the skeletal changes to accommodate that weight. These mechanisms constitute the body's reference system, the checks and balances by which it maintains itself within narrow limits. Whatever amount of fat you maintain for a period of a year or more becomes *the* reference amount for the body's defenses. The body constantly monitors these fat stores with hormonal messengers, such as glycerol, which flow in the bloodstream to the brain-monitoring system. The bloodstream level is exactly in proportion to the fat store. We call this the *fatpoint.*

The fatpoint is an implacable foe of dieters. The body defends its fat cells against invasion and deprivation just as it defends all its other cells. Whenever there is a sudden change, a crash diet, for example, as fat stores begin to be depleted, the body sets in motion all sorts of powerful mechanisms to return to its fatpoint.[19] It reduces metabolism, burning calories more slowly, making you slow and drowsy. It restricts available glycogen use, making you weak and irritable. It increases digestive efficiency, grabbing every calorie that passes, making more calories bioavailable than normally. (Consequently, eating less food does not necessarily mean fewer bioavailable calories.) Finally, it sensitizes all the powerful mechanisms of eyes, nose, mouth and stomach to respond to the sight, smell, taste and bulk of food. Inevitably, the usual forms of dieting simply set you up for binging.

If you have been overweight for a year or more, your body demands to be kept at that fatpoint. So ordinary dieting just can't work. Dr. Jeffrey Flier at Harvard, for example, found that twenty-three obese people lost a whopping average of 18 percent of body weight while on a supervised diet. But their enzyme levels correlated with their fatpoints. During the diet, enzyme levels remained almost unchanged, just waiting to put the fat back on again.[20] So you can wire up your mouth, empty the fridge, and run a treadmill to exhaustion. Temporarily, you may lose twenty pounds a week. But all the body machinery is just waiting for your first good meal after the diet. All the enzymes are ready to convert every calorie to fat. All the capillaries, built over years to nourish fat stores, are waiting to grab every molecule. You can't win. Crash diets have been found a total failure for long-term weight control.[21] In fact, 95 percent of *all* diets bring nothing but a very temporary and uncomfortable dip in the bathroom scale.[22] Even then, the short-term success of many fad diets probably relies on the recommended food being so disgusting that you can't bear to eat it.

Dieting Usually Makes You Fatter

Reliable studies show that it takes years to get fat.[23] Once you are fat, however, and have been for some time, the body slowly adjusts all its defense mechanisms to the new weight, and you have a new fatpoint. The body resists any attempts to change this new fatpoint. If you eat little, as many fat people do in an attempt to lose weight, all the defenses are continually activated. The body conserves its fat like gold.

Many diet books, both professional and popular, insist that fat people differ fundamentally from slim people. Some claim fatties don't have to eat much to stay fat. Others claim they can lose fat more easily because they have more of it. The error is in measuring the dynamics of people who are already overweight, instead of how they got to that state. Metabolic derangements found in the obese are mostly a consequence of the fat, not a cause of it.[24]

It's no mystery how a fat body maintains all that flesh on the same food that sustains a thin body. The answer lies mainly in the nature of fat cells. They are much less active metabolically than other cells.[25] Fat stores burn little energy. A man who is half composed of fat at 300 pounds total weight doesn't need any more food than someone of 180 pounds who is all muscle. As the amount of fat increases relative to muscle, the overall metabolic rate of the body declines. Fatties burn far fewer calories per pound than people of normal weight. So the fat body is much less affected by dieting. But not because of an inborn defect, only because of the fat it has accumulated.

With multiple bodily controls holding weight at the fatpoint, why do we get fat at all? There are two main reasons. The first is continual overeating of rubbish. As we have seen, much American food is nutritionally valueless. So we are contantly triggering the body defenses to demand more nutrients. So it constantly programs the appetite to overeat. The fatpoint is edged very gradually upward, because the overeating, in a vain bid for nutrition, puts the usual weight on the high side of fatpoint most of the time. Until the body is adequately nourished, you are fighting a losing battle with fat.

You need gain only one ounce a week to be 3¼ pounds heavier in a year. We know the fatpoint will shift that much. In the twenty years from age twenty to age forty, you can quietly gain sixty-five pounds, and skeleton, muscles, glands and enzymes will all have adjusted to suit. Your fatpoint has then shifted up sixty-five pounds, and the body will resist vigorously any attempts to lower it. So runs the course of middle-aged spread. There is no natural spread with aging, only the middle-aged result of years of overeating.

The second way we gain weight is by repeated dieting. Whenever you abandon a diet, rebound overeating carries your weight beyond the fatpoint, while body defenses are still mobilized from the dieting to protect the fat store. You might think that alternative mechanisms should come into play as soon as the body detects more fat than the accustomed level. But unfortunately, there are competing body mechanisms that prevent this from happening just long enough for you to gain a few pounds. These mechanisms are stronger than the fatpoint controls because they protect against life-threatening situations. They are the body's defenders of its overall nutritional state.

Complete vitamin and mineral supplements are especially important for dieters. Their bodies are frequently badly malnourished, not only by the junk foods that put on their fat, but also by the fad diets with which they try to take it off. We cannot find a single popular diet that offers optimum nutrition. So most people who abandon diets are already malnourished. Then, the first thing they do is dig into processed carbohydrates to get the quick satisfaction of sugar. As we have seen, *all* these edibles contain very few nutrients. So, even when weight rises above the fatpoint, nutrition controls override the fatpoint controls and keep the appetite primed for continued eating. The *net* effect of the diet is to shift the usual weight *up*. When it has been held up for a while, the fatpoint edges up also. So dieting can easily make you fatter than if you never did it.

Four attempts at dieting a year, the average number for overweight people who come to our clinics, may shift the fatpoint upwards by eight to sixteen pounds. So the net result of all that dieting effort can be a considerable *gain* in weight. Against this knowledge, to severely restrict the food of obese people is absurd. It sets the body's defenses going full steam ahead. All it accomplishes is to make them miserable. The short-term weight loss is inevitably followed by immediate weight gain to a higher level than before. With the methods of control of overweight now in common use, even in hospitals, correction of obesity is virtually hopeless.[26] If you are seriously overweight, give this chapter to your physician. It will be another ten years before the information is disseminated through medical journals.

You CAN Fight Fat and Win

The more fiercely you diet, the more fiercely the body protects its fatpoint. You can't beat it with willpower for long. But you can win, and win permanently, by cooperating with your body. The only long-term effective method of weight loss is to change the body's reference system so that the fatpoint is lowered. This requires careful programming. Unless the body is adequately nourished, you will not be able to stop overeating.

So, first you have to obtain a complete vitamin and mineral supplement to shut down the body's malnourishment defenses. Then you can begin to reduce calories. But you must not reduce them so much that they trigger the fatpoint defenses. If you do, the whole cycle of metabolic shutdown and appetite explosion begins anew. We have found that two hundred to five hundred calories a day is the maximum you can reduce below *your* usual amount of food without triggering the defenses. Particular calorie levels given by diets are useless. The reduction must be in relation to *your* eating pattern.

Such a reduction yields a *maximum* weight loss of between one-half pound and one pound a week. Gradually, over the course of a year, the fatpoint edges down as the body remodels itself around the new usual weight, always a little on the low side of the existing fatpoint. The minor change in calories slips by the fatpoint defenses, and the supplements keep the nutrition defenses quiet. Within a year you lose between twenty-five and fifty pounds. But the great difference between this loss and most other losses by dieting is that ravenous hunger, binging, sickness, nausea and all the other hazards of dieting do not occur. With normal cell turnover the body slowly adapts its enzyme levels, its muscles, its skeleton, its glands, to the new, lower weight. The fatpoint drops to suit.

In one study at the University of Auckland we followed the progress of two women about fifteen to twenty pounds overweight who decided to crash-diet, buddy-style, to fashionable slender. We compared these two women with two others, about thirty pounds overweight, who started our optimum-nutrition weight-loss program. Over twelve months the weights of the two crash dieters oscillated like the proverbial yo-yo. At the end, one was five pounds lighter, the other two pounds heavier than when they began, after a lot of fruitless hunger, irritability and self-denial. Does it sound familiar? In contrast, one of the women following our program lost seventeen pounds, the other twenty-three pounds. Neither reported any undesirable effects. So don't count calories, count optimum nutrition.

One or two tricks can help you along. The taste, smell and sight of food are appetitive stimuli which naturally trigger eating responses. In our evolutionary past they formed part of nutritive foods and ensured that we ate the right ones. Now, technology has enabled us to remove appetitive stimuli, such as sweetness, from nutritive contexts in fruits and vegetables, and put them into edibles that don't deserve the name of food. Our inherited appetites still react to the old stimuli, but today they tempt us continually to eat rubbish. It's fair to say that eighty million fat Americans are waddling testimony to the power of food technology to turn them into carbohydrate-processing plants to line food manufacturers' pockets. So it's a good idea to keep the rubbish as far away from you as possible.

Appetitive mechanisms are not turned off by junk food, because it lacks the nutrients to satisfy them. So we constantly tend to overeat, as the body drives us on in a vain bid for nourishment. Individually designed vitamin and mineral supplements correct this tendency by providing the missing nutrition. What they don't correct is our habits. Professor Stanley Schachter and his colleagues have shown repeatedly that overweight people have learned to react almost automatically to sights, sounds, smells, even pictures and descriptions of food.[27] To counteract this conditioning, it makes sense not to keep stacks of ice cream, candy, cookies and soft drinks in the house. It makes sense to have the picture of TV health guru Richard Simmons saying "Naughty, naughty" taped on the fridge door. It makes sense to keep a supply of fresh crudités and bowls of fruit on hand. And it also makes sense to reward your weight loss with presents and trips.

But the negative cues beloved of some psychologists are nonsense. Weighing yourself daily, standing naked in front of the mirror, your full-length photo on the wall to gag over, time-locks on the fridge, filling the house with grapefruit—these just set you up for frustration and failure. So do calorie charts and lists of low-cal foods. They only increase external cues for eating. Every time you consult one, you are exposing yourself to food cues and *increasing* your desire to eat. Remember, as we discussed in Chapter 3, one binge a week will not hurt, especially if you binge on a set day, such as every Saturday. It will do wonders to keep the psychological wolves at bay. Of course, when you have lost twenty-five pounds, the full-length mirror and scales start to become rewards too.

Another trick which works in our clinics and for other scientists is to put patients on a high-fiber diet. High-fiber foods, such as fruits, vegetables, whole grains, brown rice and nuts, subdue appetitive responses. The mechanisms of mouth and throat are tamed by the extra chewing and swallowing required. The stomach is tamed by the extra bulk.[28] High-fiber foods confer two other benefits especially for the overweight. First, they do wonders for regularity. Second, controlled trials show they reduce the incidence of hemorrhoids.

The final trick is exercise. But throw away any books that show you how many calories are used by this or that type of activity. Weight lost through exercise has nothing to do with the calories used up by doing it. The trick is that brisk, aerobic exercise for thirty minutes or more raises the body's metabolic rate for up to fifteen hours afterward.[29] You don't have to huff your heart out either. A brisk walk is every bit as good as jogging or sweating at a gym class. Better, because there is little risk of injury, it is far more comfortable to do and it fits more easily into a normal working day. So you are more likely to keep it up. "Dropout" describes 95 percent of people who take on strenuous exercise programs.

One study with mildly overweight middle-aged men showed that a program of light jogging and nothing else reduced weight by an average of 10.1 pounds. All the weight lost was fat, measured accurately. The calories used by the exercise itself counted for only about three pounds of the decrease.[30]

Because each bout of exercise speeds metabolism, the frequency of exercising is also important. Well-known authority Dr. Leonard Epstein has shown that people who exercise five days a week lose twice as much weight as those who exercise three days a week. Once-a-week exercising has *no* effect on weight loss, no matter how long the session.[31] Below a certain frequency, the metabolism-speeding effect seems to be overcome by other bodily mechanisms.

There is even more value in frequent exercise if it is done in conjunction with a modest reduction in calories. Reducing food intake, no matter how carefully done, always carries the risk of a defensive metabolic slowdown and appetite explosion, triggered by the body's fatpoint monitors. Exercising daily counteracts this tendency by keeping you on a metabolic high.

Because of your past experiences with exercise, you may be reading this with disbelief. The main reason exercise fails in many weight-loss schemes is poor nutrition. Every step you jog increases your body's needs for nutrients. Without them, exercise simply puts an additional load on a system already likely to be malnourished before the dieting, and by the diet itself. Under such circumstances exercise can and does result in serious illness. So do not try it without a complete, individual vitamin and mineral supplement.

Finally, when you exercise, please cooperate with nature. The human body evolved to run on the soft, yielding surfaces of forests and plains. That is what the skeleton is designed to withstand. Only in the last few hundred years has it faced a lifetime of absorbing the shocks to feet, ankles, knees and backs caused by constant pounding on hard surfaces like wood, tarmac and concrete. No wonder it buckles under the strain. The average urban dweller can't avoid hard surfaces. So, whenever you exercise, especially if you are heavy, you must carry the soft surface around with you, in the form of properly padded sports shoes designed for shocks, like the New Balance 720 and 900 series running shoes. Tennis shoes will not do at all. And bare feet are worse. Don't even dance on gym floors in bare feet. It may look wonderful, but it's hell on your skeleton. The woodland nymphs danced on the leaves. If you can't afford the supershoes, at least insert effective shock-absorbing insoles like Spenco or Sorbothane in your gym shoes. Without them, your exercise, even brisk walking, can turn into a skeletal disaster.

Over the last nine years we have applied the principles described in this chapter to many stubborn cases of overweight. Our success rate is 80 percent. Not the short-term weight loss falsely claimed as success by most weight-loss programs. We have followed our clients for up to eight years now. Eight out of every ten who have remained on the supplements continue to control their weight without difficulty. Now they can enjoy a Knickerbocker Sundae without anxiety—and not gain an ounce.

CHAPTER 9

PREVENTING CARDIOVASCULAR DISEASE

CHANCES ARE YOU WILL suffer cardiovascular disease and have begun to develop it already. Chances are you have been grossly misinformed of the risk factors in this development by media reports and advertising. This chapter corrects the misinformation and gives you the evidence that prevention of cardiovascular disease is possible by avoiding bodily pollution and improving individual nutrition.

How Many of Us?

Hypertension (high blood pressure) is the forerunner of much cardiovascular disease. One in every five adults has this disorder, which grows so progressively worse with age that life-insurance companies allow some extent of raised blood pressure to be counted as normal in older people.[1] Yet hypertension is not a natural effect of aging. Some countries do not have the disease at all. Therefore, it is preventable.

Hypertension combines with heart and blood vessel degeneration to put thirty million Americans in the throes of manifest cardiovascular disease. In 1977, a typical year, it killed over a million of them, who were promptly replaced by over a million new cases.[2] Hypertension and arteriosclerosis (thickening and loss of elasticity in the artery walls) are the triggering conditions that have left two million Americans incapacitated by strokes, and that kill two hundred thousand stroke victims each year. They are also major causes of the million-plus heart attacks each year which kill seven hundred thousand of their unfortunate recipients. The worst of these statistics is that sixty thousand people a year are dying of heart disease between the ages of thirty-five and fifty-five, when they should be enjoying the prime of life. A quarter of all people killed by cardiovascular disease have not reached age sixty-five.[3]

Only a minority of sufferers are aware that they have hypertension or arteriosclerosis,[4] and fewer do anything to prevent these preventable conditions. Even after developing to a noticeable degree, they can be arrested, controlled and sometimes reversed. But after the trauma of heart attack or stroke, medicine can often do little but comfort the patient's remaining days. A visit to a hospital for victims of cardiovascular trauma offers abundant grisly evidence that prevention is the only road.

Degeneration Is Occurring Earlier

We must get rid of the myth that cardiovascular diseases are rampant today only because science saves us from infectious diseases, so that we get old enough for our hearts and arteries to wear out. If so, then the incidence of cardiovascular diseases would be similar throughout developed countries. It is not. By middle age, Americans have *nine times* as much heart disease as the Japanese,[5] and it begins much earlier in life. Autopsies performed on American soldiers killed in action in Vietnam showed that one in every two already had arteriosclerosis. The average age of these youths was twenty-two years![6] These young soldiers would be fitter and healthier than the national average for their age. So, if they are degenerating, what is happening to the rest of us? Autopsies done in Japan on the same age group rarely find arteriosclerosis.[7] Autopsies done on American soldiers in the Second World War showed much less arteriosclorosis.[8] Today it is likely that half of America's young men already have the beginnings of heart disease.

This awful precursor of heart attacks and strokes is now turning up in our children. In a study in New Orleans, the fatty streaks and intermediate lesions that precede atherosclerotic plaques were found in the aortas of almost all children aged ten years or older.[9] So, even if adults are not concerned enough to prevent cardiovascular disease in themselves, they should at least be concerned that their children reach adulthood without it.

The same sad tale attends hypertension. Australia and New Zealand, for example, have the same rising blood pressure with age that has become endemic in America, including the state of Hawaii. Yet in some of the Pacific Islands that border Australia, New Zealand and Hawaii, there is no rise in blood pressure with age. Even late in life, hypertension is very rare there.[10] Different races of people, you might argue. Not the answer. When Pacific Islanders emigrate to New Zealand, within a few years their blood pressure starts to rise. The more they adopt the Western lifestyle of processed foods, overeating, little exercise, bodily pollution and poor nutrition, the earlier hypertension appears.[11] What we are unknowingly doing to our bodies and those of our children is killing us and them earlier in life than tuberculosis killed our great-grandkin in 1900. Preventable heart disease is turning the terribly young into the chronically infirm, insidiously destroying the body and brain power essential to the continuing progress of the nation.

Limits of Medicine

Even the tiniest bit of heart disease eventually becomes physically obvious. Once it does, medicine can often do naught but help you live ill longer. Heart transplants, triple bypasses and pacemakers are wonderful tributes to the progressive skill of our simian fingers. But only the very rare patient undergoing these ministrations ever golfs, swims, rides or even jumps for joy again (except as a two-minute media whiz with a resuscitator standing by).

Television soap operas fool us that the shining machines and syncopated beeps of coronary care units could breathe life into a garden gnome. In fact, Dr. W. G. Mather and many colleagues, in an extensive study for the British Ministry of Health, showed that these wildly expensive units do not lengthen the lives or reduce the disability of heart-attack victims any more than simple treatment at home by their general practitioner.[12] With or without space-age life supports, you are just as likely to die of a stroke as was your great-grandfather in 1900.[13]

Neither are drugs the sure answer. Humbug apologists for the drug industry would make P. T. Barnum blush with their cholesterol sideshow. Suspecting the trumpery, the National Heart, Lung and Blood Institute mounted the Coronary Drug Project to examine whether cholesterol-lowering drugs actually do reduce heart disease. Most have now been shown to be ineffective. The worst finding is that some drugs, namely dextrothyroxine and the conjugated estrogens, while they do lower cholesterol, actually *increase* the progress of heart disease. Between 20 percent and 30 percent *more* people die on these prescribed poisons than if given no treatment at all.[14]

Medical professionals readily admit to each other that therapy for heart disease is only marginally effective. We can hardly blame *them.* By the time the disease shows itself, physicians are faced with hearts and blood vessels that have suffered years of maltreatment at the hands of their owners. When therapy does work, it often depends more on how patients change their lifestyle than on any medical maneuvers.[15] Avoiding further bodily pollution and improving nutrition and exercise are often the crucial determinants.

If you live that long. Remember, cardiovascular disease is a systemic degeneration that progresses for years without symptoms. If you pollute and malnourish your body into disease, don't expect your doctor to spot impending disaster. His first and only indication may be the description on your death certificate. Dr. Lewis Kuller studied 1,857 people who died in the course of a year in the city of Baltimore.[16] These people were not elderly. All of them were between twenty and sixty-four years of age. One in every three died suddenly, unexpectedly, and over half the deaths were from cardiovascular disease. Eighty-six of them had been seen by a physician within seven days before death, and 326 had been seen by a physician within the six months prior to death. Some had known heart disease, but not a single one was expected to die. Ninety of the victims fulfilled all the criteria of the study for good health!

Hypertension Kills

Hypertension is such a silent killer that only one in ten Americans who have the problem is even aware of it. Just like arteriosclerosis, hypertension may progressively disease your body for many years without evincing a single noticeable symptom to warn you. This hidden degeneration is a major health problem in America. Dr. Robert Levy, director of the National Heart, Lung and Blood Institute, puts hypertension as *the* Number 1 risk factor for strokes and heart attacks.[17] If you don't even know you have it, you certainly cannot prevent them.

In America, Britain and most Westernized countries, after age twenty-five blood pressure rises steadily, so you cannot rely on readings taken way back. In five years your pressure could rise from normal (120/80 plus or minus 10 mm Hg) to the pathological level of 160/95 mm Hg. Today thirty-five million Americans have this degree of hypertension, and most do not know it. They have quadrupled their risk of stroke and doubled their risk of heart attack.[18] Another twenty-five million have borderline hypertension, 140/90–160/95 mm Hg. So, together, sixty million Americans are at risk.

As most sufferers are blissfully unaware of their condition, they do not seek medical aid. Unless a physician can confront the disease, clearly medicine can do nothing. Many people know they should have checkups but naturally avoid the time, trouble and expense of visits to a doctor with the chance of being told they are ill when they feel perfectly healthy. So it is not the physicians' problem. Fortunately, there is a simple solution to knowing whether or not you have hypertension. For the cost of one medical visit you can buy a blood-pressure measuring instrument (sphygmomanometer) sold in many electronics stores. With this small but wise investment you can measure the whole family as many times as you like for years. (If you do find high blood pressure, *then* see your physician.) This simple device is your first step in prevention of progressive hypertension.

The second step is to know what causes it. A popular myth is that high blood pressure is a natural effect of aging, not of our nutrition or lifestyle. Not so. Many populations do not have the disease at all. They retain a constant 120/80 plus or minus 10 mm Hg throughout life, and they have many fewer deaths from cardiovascular disease.[19] These populations vary widely in culture, lifestyle and diet. They range from Mayan Indian hill farmers through Cook Islanders of the Pacific to Masai tribesmen and Somali nomads. From comparisons of these groups with each other and with Western society we know that smoking, alcohol, salt, fats, obesity and exercise are all involved in hypertension. We know also that where there is hypertension, atherosclerosis is likely also.[20]

But these variables together offer only a partial explanation. A major factor linking all the nonhypertensive societies is that their cultures are stable, the role and status of each person are well defined, and traditional values are honored. In contrast, all Westernized societies are characterized by fragmented roles, status conflicts, rejection of traditional values and constantly changing rules, all of which make life very uncertain.[21]

This has a lot to do with hypertension. We forget that our physiology is little more advanced than that of an ape. We have inherited many inborn reactions which are more appropriate to our gibbering ancestors, which belong in a world where survival depended on the ability to fight or flee. This fight/flight reaction occurs automatically in the face of any threatening situation. It is a coordinated visceral, hormonal and muscular discharge pattern. One component is the raised blood pressure necessary for the violent muscular activity of fighting or running away.

Western society is unsuited to such a reaction tendency for two reasons. First, the number of threat situations is vastly increased because of the uncertainties and conflicts described above. So we get more than our share of fight/flight reactions. Second, we are socially conditioned not to fight or to run away but to stay still, even though physiologically boiling. The muscular component of the fight/flight reaction is inhibited by your social learning that the right to swing your fist stops where the next fellow's nose begins. So the metabolic and cardiovascular resources mobilized by the fight/flight reaction are not used in the way prescribed by our inherited physiology. Blood pressure stays up because there is none of the increased blood flow through muscle blood vessels that occurs with violent activity to reduce the pressure. Oft repeated, these transient increases in blood pressure are the probable basis of much permanent hypertension.[22] Next time you fall victim to a cacophony of rush-hour car horns, glance in your mirror to see blood pressure putting its tracery on your eyeballs, sure evidence of our evolutionary incapacity to adapt to the stress of urban living.

But if the reactions are automatic, what can be done to prevent them? There are two avenues. First, recent studies have shown that relaxation training, although difficult, will reduce stress reactions, including the blood-pressure component.[23] Success is also possible in learning to lower blood pressure with a biofeedback device that tells you minute by minute your pressure level. With extensive biofeedback training, even people with pathological hypertension can learn to reduce it.[24] So it is possible to modify the automatic reactions.

Most of us, however, have neither the time nor the patience to learn these techniques. Fortunately, the second approach is much simpler. By avoiding bodily pollution and improving nutrition, we can make the body stronger and therefore resistant to the damaging effects of elevations of blood pressure. We can also lower basal blood pressure, that is, the level of blood pressure when not under stress. If this is low, then the effects of the transient rises of fight/flight responses are also diminished. For it is the force of the pressure peak on the artery which is likely the damaging agent.[25] The higher the peak, the worse the damage. Similarly, we can also inhibit development of atherosclerosis, which again assists in keeping blood pressure stable. Let us look first at bodily pollution.

Smoking Breeds Cardiovascular Disease

The primary pollutant today is undoubtedly smoking. Despite the understandable publicity efforts of the tobacco industry, the connection between smoking and cancer is now irrefutable. Less well known is the equally strong link between smoking and cardiovascular disease. Smoking one pack of cigarettes a day gives you twice the risk of heart attack and five times the risk of stroke of a nonsmoker.[26] Each year in Britain, thirty thousand people die of heart disease as a direct result of smoking. Between the ages of thirty-five and forty-five, when people should be hale and healthy, smoking two packs or more a day makes you five times more likely to die of heart disease. In America a huge study of U.S. veterans found the same fivefold risk between ages thirty-five and forty-five, with a jump to ten times the death risk between ages forty-five and fifty-five.[27]

Don't believe you dodge it if you are young, watch your diet, keep trim and exercise regularly. As long as you smoke, cardiovascular disease is growing silently in your body. For some years I interviewed young heart-attack and stroke victims, vainly trying to discover why the trauma had occurred. Apart from a common habit of smoking, there seemed to be no reason, no illness, no sudden stress, no family or other disaster. Before the attack many were fit and healthy and had recent physicals showing nothing abnormal. Yet in a few horrific minutes their bodies had been irreversibly damaged. At the time I had insufficient evidence to implicate smoking, but now the mystery is solved. Dr. W. J. McKenna, among others, has shown that young people with a completely healthy cardiovascular profile can easily have heart attacks or strokes, because *smoking increases the tendency of the blood to clot.*[28]

Two major pollutants in smoking which affect the cardiovascular system are nicotine and carbon monoxide. Yes, carbon monoxide, the deadly gas of too many suicides. Cigarette smoke contains 3 percent to 6 percent carbon monoxide. When inhaled with air, this is diluted, but only to a level that is still eight times higher than the permissible maximum for industry. Even inhaling air polluted by smokers gives you the equivalent carbon monoxide of smoking one cigarette an hour.[29] Both carbon monoxide and nicotine increase the stickiness of platelets in the blood and facilitate the formation of clots.[30] If smoking causes pathological blood clots in young, fit people, then it is much more likely to do so in older people whose arteries are already partially blocked by atherosclerosis.

In addition, nicotine raises blood pressure and cardiac output and causes an increase in circulating fatty acids which may raise triglycerides and cholesterol in the blood.[31] High levels of both these lipids are associated with increased cardiovascular risk. Carbon monoxide also reduces blood oxygen, leading to an oxygen shortage that damages the walls of the arteries,[32] leaving them open to the formation of atherosclerotic plaques. Far more atherosclerosis is found in autopsies of smokers than nonsmokers. Nine out of every ten heavy smokers (forty or more cigarettes a day) are found to have moderate to advanced atherosclerosis compared with three out of ten nonsmokers.[33]

Once brain tissue is destroyed by a stroke, or heart muscle by a coronary, medicine can do absolutely nothing to restore it. Yet stopping smoking immediately reduces your risk. Within hours of the last cigarette, blood-clotting time returns to normal. Young or even middle-aged men who stop smoking have a major reduction in rates of cardiovascular disease compared with those who continue to smoke. Within a year of stopping, cardiovascular risk drops by half. After ten years the risk is the same as for those who have never smoked—a fitting tribute to the superb regenerative power of the human body.[34]

How difficult is it to give up smoking? Not so hard if you are really convinced. A study in Edinburgh (Scotland) showed that nearly two thirds of smokers who survived a heart attack stopped smoking immediately and were still nonsmokers a year later.[35] Also, most doctors who smoked have managed to kick the habit. If you have a doctor who still smokes, you should reject him. If he doesn't care to practice basic prevention on his own health, he may not care to practice it on yours.

In stroke wards it is heartrending to see the needless, senseless waste of human potential in smokers left paralyzed, blind, or reduced to permanent daydreaming by the destruction of their brains. By their own puffs these unfortunates are condemned to a living hell. The only reason this destructive habit remains legal, despite overwhelming evidence that it kills millions each year, is that governments seldom judge it reasonable to inhibit evils that are the highly taxable work of powerful, self-righteous segments of industry. Future historians will look back in bewilderment at a nation clever enough on the one hand to make heroin illegal in 1912 because of its effects on health, but stupid enough on the other hand to keep using tobacco in increasing quantities for the rest of the century.

Cholesterol

The public is fed such a deluge of hogwash on the dangers of cholesterol that a separate section is needed to refute it. Cholesterol is a fatlike steroid alcohol essential to the healthy operation of the human body. It has important functions in the synthesis of the steroid hormones and is a precursor of the bile acids. It forms part of every organ, including the brain, the heart, even the skin. *Most* cholesterol in the body is made there in the liver. Despite Madison Avenue's concerted cries of "wolf," only a small amount of cholesterol is absorbed from the diet.[36] The internally made cholesterol can deposit as plaques in the arteries just as easily as dietary cholesterol.

Medical science has firmly established that the high cholesterol counts found in atherosclerosis are a result of complex disorders of lipid metabolism and artery wall damage, *not* a result of any cholesterol you put in your mouth.[37] A high cholesterol count is only one symptom of a widespread disorder. For people with cholesterol counts within normal ranges, the body immediately reduces production of cholesterol if an excess is eaten, indicating powerful internal controls of cholesterol levels.[38] It is the disordering of these controls, not the cholesterol eaten, which gives pathological levels in the blood. After fifty years of studies, the American Heart Association has concluded that there is no proof that a low-cholesterol diet followed from early adulthood reduces the incidence of heart attacks.[39]

Cholesterol levels considered normal in medical practice vary between 125 and 240 milligrams cholesterol per 100 milliliters of blood serum (125–240 mg/dl). When calculating your own nutritional needs, you will see that I consider it better to keep your cholesterol level below 200 mg/dl. Between the commonly accepted levels, additional dietary cholesterol in a mixed diet raises blood cholesterol only a little. Even two eggs a day, long held as villains in heart disease, raise cholesterol by only 5–12 mg/dl. One egg a day has no effect at all, even in subjects with cholesterol counts over 200 mg/dl.[40]

Cholesterol levels above 240 mg/dl increase your risk of cardiovascular trauma by three times, and by six times if over 260 mg/dl. So, if—and only if—your level is high, it is prudent to avoid pushing it up even a bit by eating large amounts of high-cholesterol foods. In order of cholesterol content, high-cholesterol foods are eggs, poultry livers, dairy products and organ meats.

The most drastic way to lower cholesterol is by long-term use of drugs. With devilish cunning and monumental ignorance of the complexity of cholesterol metabolism, the drug industry has clung to the claim that cholesterol-lowering drugs reduce cardiovascular disease. The nationwide Coronary Drug Project, however, using 8,341 patients, aged thirty to sixty-four, has shown that most of the drugs don't work. Worse, some of them kill more patients than they cure. A pertinent example is dextrothyroxine, a thyroid hormone analogue. Over five years this drug lowered cholesterol an average of 12 percent—not a huge drop. A man at 265 mg/dl would go down to 233 mg/dl, still at risk. The effect on health was huge, though. Nearly a fifth *more* patients died on the drug than in the control group given no drugs at all. In addition, dextrothyroxine pushed other biochemical and hematologic (blood) indices outside normal limits, caused toxic reactions, pain and discomfort and abnormal liver function.[41]

Although they may be useful in short-term intervention, the awful side effects of long-term use of all cholesterol-lowering drugs is a 100 percent indication that they radically disorder bodily processes. After the horror-story reports of their effects in the *Journal of the American Medical Association,* I must give wholehearted praise to the director of the National Heart, Lung and Blood Institute, Dr. Robert Levy, for his recent emphasis that "diet is the cornerstone of therapy."[42]

If dietary cholesterol itself is only a minor contributor to hypercholesterolemia, as it is called in jargonese, then clearly you can't do much by cutting *it* out of your diet. Another popular dietary maneuver is to substitute PUFAs, or polyunsaturated fatty acids, for animal fats. Alas, unsaturated fats lower cholesterol levels only under very specialized dietary conditions. Professor Roger Williams, in an excellent review of the evidence, indicates how a high-PUFA diet can *increase* blood-cholesterol level, or in other conditions can lower it, but only by depositing the excess cholesterol in the liver and muscles. Increasing your intake of PUFAs may also accelerate thrombus formation and atherosclerosis and cause a Vitamin E deficiency.[43] It is a dangerous practice subtly foisted on the public and gullible physicians by commercial interests. In 1950 PUFAs were only 2 percent of the American diet. By 1970 they had risen to 6 percent. If they helped, we should have seen a reduction in cardiovascular disease. Instead, it increased steadily over the whole twenty years.[44]

A much better way of avoiding animal fats is to replace meat protein in the diet. Regular eating of soybeans, for example, reduces cholesterol substantially in people with high levels, and even in people with levels in the range accepted as normal (125–240 mg/dl).[45] Another sure way to reduce cholesterol, as Professor Ancel Keys has shown, is to eat less meat and more complex carbohydrates, such as brown rice and legumes (peas and beans).[46]

Not quite so effective but still very useful if you must have those steaks, is to increase the pectin in your diet. Pectin is a complex carbohydrate found in fruit and vegetables. Pectin reliably lowers cholesterol in experimental animals and in human volunteers, again even when the levels are within the American norm. No one knows exactly how it works, but pectin binds with substances necessary to carry cholesterol in the bloodstream, making them unavailable as carriers. Hence, cholesterol declines.[47] You can obtain pectin either as a supplement or by eating raw fruits and vegetables, especially grapefruit, oranges, lemons, apples and carrots.

Another effective dietary tactic is to use lecithin supplements. Lecithin is not a crank health food as many people think, but is an essential substance manufactured in the human body. It forms part of your nerves and your liver and is a major constituent of your cell membranes. In the blood it acts partly as a lubricant and partly as an emulsifier, dissolving and reducing the size of cholesterol particles and easing their passage through the system. The blood level of this benevolent phospholipid can be increased easily by dietary lecithin. An ounce a day reliably lowers cholesterol,[48] and if you don't want to take supplements, soybeans are a good food source.

Saturated Fat Pollution

You can also lower cholesterol by reducing saturated fats in the diet, by eating less meat, especially pork, bacon and ham, and fewer dairy products, and by trimming off meat fat before cooking. In Western society, though mysteriously not in some primitive societies, high-fat diets are strongly correlated with high cholesterol levels and cardiovascular disease.[49] To understand why, we have to step a mite further into medical science. In order to flow in the bloodstream, the otherwise insoluble cholesterol has to become bound to a class of proteins (lipoproteins) of two main types: high-density and low-density. The low-density lipoproteins (LDLs) carry 60 percent to 75 percent of blood cholesterol. It is their concentration in the blood, therefore, that largely determines cholesterol level, and is directly associated with cardiovascular disease.[50] Instead of hypercholesterolemia, the new jargon word is hyperlipoproteinemia.

High-density lipoproteins (HDLs) normally carry 25 percent of the blood cholesterol, but much less if you have high cholesterol. At high cholesterol levels the high-density lipoproteins are too low and the low-density lipoproteins are too high. The world-famous Framingham study, in which the whole population of Framingham in Massachusetts has been intensively studied for many years, has shown recently that increased high-density lipoproteins reduce cardiovascular risk.[51] High-density lipoprotein seems to act as a benevolent scavenger, removing cholesterol deposits from artery walls and promoting their return to the liver to be excreted as bile.

One way to protect your high-density lipoprotein level stems from the recent discovery that it is correlated with plasma Vitamin C level.[52] The higher the C, the higher the high-density lipoprotein. Individual needs vary widely, but you can determine your need for Vitamin C by working through the system in Chapter 6.

Another astonishing discovery is that *moderate* alcohol consumption increases high-density lipoproteins.[53] It is also correlated with reduced atherosclerosis and reduced cardiovascular risk.[54] Moderate means two ounces a day, that is, two beers or two glasses of wine or two shots of hard liquor. Beyond this level the effect disappears. It was hard to decide to recommend this tactic, because the existence of America's seventeen million alcoholics indicates that many people can't stop at two drinks. Overconsumption of alcohol damages both heart muscle and heart rhythm. Nevertheless, the evidence is firm. A daily sip protects you.

You can also lower low-density lipoproteins to reduce cardiovascular risk. The best method is to restrict saturated fats in the diet.[55] Apart from drugs, the only other established method is the use of Vitamin B_3 in nicotinic-acid form, which lowers low-density lipoproteins by inhibiting production of their precursor in the liver.[56] And as an unexpected bonus, B_3 also raises high-density lipoprotein levels, though no one knows why. None of the lipid-lowering drugs raise high-density lipoprotein levels.[57] In healthy people amounts of nicotinic acid over 100 mg a day should not be used except under medical supervision. For people with known high cholesterol or lipoprotein fraction disorders, ask your physician about treatment with this vitamin. It is approved for this use by the National Institutes of Health.

Excessive saturated fats in the diet do more than disrupt cholesterol and other lipid metabolism. To understand the devious ways they work their evils, we need another snippet of science. Atherosclerosis and clot formation in the bloodstream are not independent. Clots—or thrombi, to be accurate—are likely a major cause of atherosclerotic plaques.[58] A thrombus starts with the clumping of platelets in the bloodstream. This activity also damages the artery walls,[59] providing the lesions that cholesterol can enter to form plaques. Saturated fats increase the tendency of platelets to clump and blood to clot,[60] thereby increasing both arterial damage and atherosclerosis. Recent, superb studies in France and Britain by Dr. S. Renaud and his colleagues of the

French National Institute of Health and Medical Research show that reducing saturated fats in the diet also reduces both clumping and clotting in the arteries.[61] So, take the grilled salmon over the filet mignon every time.

Moderate alcohol consumption (2 oz a day) also reduces platelet clumping.[62] If your attitude to "moderate" is too elastic, then dietary garlic works as well. Yes, plain old garlic reduces platelet clumping. Not an old wives tale, but now measured in recent controlled studies.[63] The active substance in garlic is the essential oil methyl allyl trisulphide. Onions have a similar effect,[64] probably because of the oil allyl propyl disulphide. Unlike alcohol, there are no undesirable effects with onions and garlic (apart from social isolation). I cannot recommend specific amounts, because essential oil content varies widely with type, quality and storage time. Simply eat them fresh and freely for a healthier cardiovascular system—and more room in elevators.

Another common substance that reduces platelet clumping, and lowers cholesterol and other undesirable lipid fractions, is dietary calcium. This effect is found even in young adults, who are unlikely to be calcium deficient.[65] Older people, who are often calcium deficient, are likely to show even better responses. Dietary calcium also offsets the effects of saturated fats in the diet.[66] Calcium in the water supply is thought to be one of the major protective minerals against heart disease. Communities with hard water (high calcium and magnesium) consistently have less heart disease than soft-water communities.[67] You can calculate your need for calcium using the system in Chapter 6.

Sugar: White, Brown, Raw, All Deadly

Controversy waxes and wanes, but no one can refute Professor John Yudkin's twenty years of findings that excess sugar consumption is correlated with heart attacks and atherosclerosis.[68] Four ounces of sugar a day over a long period is enough to put you at high risk. Most Americans eat more. And yet we puzzle over our heart-disease problem! Saving graces are low blood cholesterol and a slim body. Such people are highly resistant to the bad effects of sugar because they metabolize it efficiently. Not so fatties with high cholesterol counts. In these unfortunates dietary sugar ends up as free fatty acids which boost low-density lipoproteins to dangerous levels.[69] Enough said. We return again and again to the destructive actions of sugar in the chapters on diabetes, obesity and food pollution. For health of the heart and blood vessels alone, keep your sugar below three ounces a day.

And that includes all the hocus-pocus raw sugars, brown sugars, turbinado sugars, honeys, molasses and fructoses invested with magical properties by health-food hucksters manipulating your sweet tooth. They are all the same as far as the cardiovascular system is concerned. Remember too that sugar is now being added to everything from bread to pâté. You don't have to eat candy bars to get excess sugar.

Salt 'n' Soda: Both White and Deadly

In some ways salt is worse than sugar. It is the sodium in sodium chloride, our common table salt, that is the culprit. The sodium in baking soda is just as bad. Other sources of sodium are indigestion remedies and soft drinks. Not only does sodium disorder lipid metabolism,[70] but in many people it also raises blood pressure by increasing fluid retention in the body.[71] Hence the "water pills" for hypertension.

The average American eats half an ounce of salt a day, twenty times the requirement for good nutrition.[72] You don't need to salt your food to get an excess. As discussed in Chapter 2, huge amounts of salt are added to everything from candy to frozen vegetables. That is why it's so difficult for hypertensives to keep their salt down to the 200 mg a day (just a pinch) necessary to get a good reduction in blood pressure.[73] It's certainly worthwhile to avoid obvious sources of salt, such as pickles, salt cheeses, preserved meats, canned and packeted soups, bologna, ketchup, olives, salted nuts, pretzels, saltines, salt bacon and all canned foods.

You don't have to reduce your blood pressure much to significantly reduce your risk. The National Heart, Lung and Blood Institute studied 10,940 hypertensives between 1972 and 1978. In a group with diastolic pressures between 90 and 104 mm Hg (normal is 70 to 90 mm Hg), the average reduction in pressure with drugs, diet and other advice was only 12.9 mm Hg over five years. Nevertheless, compared to a control group, deaths from stroke were reduced by 20 percent.[74] So, for even a little high blood pressure, throw away the saltcellar.

Salt substitutes are fine, especially if you are taking "water pills" (diuretics) for whatever reason. Diuretics not only remove unnecessary body sodium, but also cause a big loss of essential potassium.[75] Such a loss, left uncorrected, can cause a heart attack. Most salt substitutes are high in potassium. Don't use any of the "sea salt" preparations, no matter what they say on the labels. All are too high in sodium.

Vitamins That Promote Cardiovascular Health

At one time or other every vitamin has been touted for use in cardiovascular disease. We will consider only those few that have passed the test of rigorous experiment. The first is folic acid. Pregnant women and the elderly of both sexes are often deficient in this cofactor of the B vitamins, and it is commonly deficient in the American diet. The best sources are soybeans, liver and raw green vegetables, but cooking destroys most of the folic acid. In children a folic-acid deficiency has been associated with both congenital (present at birth) and acquired forms of heart disease.[76] Studies in animals show many deformities in the hearts and other organs of offspring of mothers who were deficient in folic acid.[77] In elderly patients with atherosclerosis blocking their arteries and folic-acid deficiency, treatment with oral folic acid has measurably improved peripheral circulation.[78]

Vitamin B_6, pyridoxine, is also associated with cardiovascular health. Most diets, as we have seen, are deficient in this vitamin. The best sources of Vitamin B_6 are sunflower seeds, wheat germ, tuna and soybeans. Monkeys made deficient in B_6 rapidly develop atherosclerosis.[79] This may be because Vitamin B_6 is used by the body in making the lecithin that is essential to normal cholesterol metabolism.

For more than forty years reports from the famous Shute Clinic in Ontario have attested to the efficacy of dietary Vitamin E supplements in a variety of heart and blood-vessel diseases. Most of these reports were case studies or small case series, culminating in a book by Dr. Wilfrid Shute, *Vitamin E for Ailing and Healthy Hearts,* in 1969. This book took the media and the public by storm, but not the medical profession. Sadly, most of Shute's findings of beneficial effects on the heart have not been supported by recent double-blind trials.[80] Vitamin E is not the magic bullet. Also, Vitamin E deficiency does not produce the clear-cut heart damage in humans that it produces in other animals. Happily, controlled studies do support Shute's work on Vitamin E treatment of peripheral vascular diseases.[81] And treatment of general atherosclerosis with Vitamin E supplements for ten years gives a higher survival rate than in patients not given this vitamin.[82]

Vitamin E has four known actions in the body which also support its use in maintaining vascular health. First, it reduces platelet clumping,[83] thereby reducing the tendency for unwanted clots to form in the arteries. Second, it is a natural anticoagulant in other ways, which prevents unwanted blood clotting, but unlike anticoagulant drugs, it does not prevent the blood clotting essential to stop the bleeding of an injury.[84] Third, adequate dietary Vitamin E is essential for normal absorption and transport of lipids (fats) in the body.[85] Fourth, it has now been demonstrated that Vitamin E increases high-density lipoprotein levels,[86] thereby reducing cardiovascular risk.

So, though it is not confirmed as benefiting the heart directly, there is little doubt of Vitamin E's value in preventing cardiovascular disease.

We have already noted the effects of Vitamin C in keeping your high-density lipoproteins high. It also helps to remove cholesterol deposits from the artery walls in animals[87] and in humans.[88] One problem in doing so in people who have atherosclerosis is that mobilizing the cholesterol deposits raises the total cholesterol in the blood, often for months. Dr. Constance Spittle, at Pinderfields Hospital in Yorkshire, England, using one gram of C daily for six weeks, found an average 10 percent *increase* in cholesterol count in atherosclerotic patients, but an 8 percent *decrease* in a control group of healthy individuals also fed the vitamin.[89] In my own cases, using apparently healthy individuals, but with cholesterol counts of 190–240 mg/dl, beneficial effects often have not appeared for three to six months. As we have seen, however, it is not a matter of Vitamin C alone, but the combination of nutrients which brings the best results.

We should note how Vitamin C works with other antioxidant nutrients to give cardiovascular protection. As we have discussed, particles called free radicals and dienes (active hydrocarbons) circulate in the human bloodstream and cause damage to the artery walls.[90] Circulating antioxidants destroy many of these particles, and therefore prevent much of the damage. The three main nutrient antioxidants are Vitamins C and E and the mineral selenium. The evidence is not strong enough to warrant using these as supplements solely for their antioxidant effects in the cardiovascular system, but combined with their other essential effects throughout the body, it is unassailable.

Minerals That Promote Cardiovascular Health

Selenium has other functions too, which are essential to cardiovascular function. This essential mineral is in short supply in the soil in many parts of the world, including ten states in

America. In these areas selenium is very low in the drinking water and in vegetables. There is now strong evidence relating this deficit to cardiovascular disease, with those in selenium-deficient areas having three times the risk.[91] In China the use of dietary selenium supplements in deficient areas has virtually eliminated a form of congestive heart disease.[92] Selenium is currently under consideration for addition to the partial list of essential nutrients that forms the Recommended Daily Allowances (RDAs) table issued by the U.S. National Research Council. Calculate your selenium requirement from the tables in Chapter 6 and keep in good heart.

Other minerals that promote cardiovascular health are calcium and magnesium. Over the last twenty years studies throughout the world have shown that "hard" water is associated with low levels of cardiovascular disease and "soft" water with high levels.[93] Coronary heart disease, hypertension and cerebrovascular disease are all affected. As even stronger evidence, if water supplies to areas are changed to become softer, then cardiovascular disease rises. If they are changed to become harder, cardiovascular disease declines.[94]

Although other minerals may be involved also, water hardness is chiefly determined by its concentrations of calcium and magnesium. The more, the harder. Hard water probably works in several ways to prevent cardiovascular disease. A most important activity occurs in your intestines. Calcium and magnesium combine with fats in the diet and make them indigestible. They are then harmlessly excreted. Another benefit is the effect in reducing the toxicity of cadmium. Cadmium is a pollutant now at high levels in all American cities. It is a suspect in our current epidemic of hypertension. Fairly low levels of cadmium in the diet can cause hypertension readily in experimental animals.[95] Hard water largely prevents this toxic effect.[96] So, if you have good hard water, be thankful. The common use of filters to remove the hardness so as to get sudsy washing water is a dreadful misapplication of science. While it gets the laundry whiter than white, it is also rotting your arteries.

A final word on minerals goes to chromium. Only recently recognized as essential for human health, this metal is another component plentiful in hard water. Recent studies show that daily supplements of 200 mcg of chromium improve the high-density lipoprotein levels even in healthy people with no hint of cardiovascular disease.[97] Chromium's importance in the prevention of human degeneration is only beginning to be appreciated.

Obesity Causes and Exercise Prevents

Good nutrition is not enough to prevent cardiovascular disease. As we saw in Chapter 8, carrying more poundage than you were designed for brings with it the twin threats of hypertension and atherosclerosis.[98] The next chapter shows how obesity is also the link between cardiovascular disease and diabetes. Staying slim is not just cosmetic vanity, it is an essential health decision.

As we saw also, exercise plays a large part in keeping the pounds away, as well as in preventing all sorts of degenerative processes in the muscles, the skeleton and the vital organs. Study is piling upon study, showing the effects of exercise on the cardiovascular system. To take a few recent examples, Drs. Dan Streja and David Mymin at the Department of Medicine of the University of Manitoba used a moderate exercise program of walking, slow jogging, stretching and light weight training three times a week with a group of thirty-two sedentary middle-aged men with coronary heart disease. Although the study was only three months long, high-density lipoproteins increased reliably, thereby reducing the risk of heart attack.[99]

You don't have to wait until you get heart disease. In another short study Dr. Sanders Williams of the Department of Medicine of Duke University showed that normal, healthy adults put on a ten-week light-exercise program significantly reduced the chances of forming unwanted clots in the bloodstream.[100] The exercise had a truly preventive effect, strengthening the system against subsequent stress.

In short-term studies the reduced risk of cardiovascular disease can only be estimated from the physiological changes. But longitudinal (long-term) studies show just how real the effects are. Just being sedentary *doubles* your risk of heart attack. In 1979 Dr. Stephen Paffenbarger reported to the American Heart Association a study on fifteen thousand college alumni who were at Harvard prior to 1950. Those who had stopped training after leaving college had much higher blood pressure,[101] and consequently much higher risk of heart attack or stroke. In a study of joggers and runners who had been exercising in this way for years, Dr. Harley Hartung at the Baylor College of Medicine showed that the greater the average distance run per week, the higher the level of protective high-density lipoproteins and the lower the level of cholesterol.[102] Both these measures indicate that jogging protects the cardiovascular system, and the farther you jog, the better.

That doesn't mean you should immediately jump into an exercise program. To the untrained body, that could be fatal. Have yourself tested first by a physician *who exercises.* If your physician doesn't exercise, then his or her knowledge of that part of preventive medicine is suspect. On receiving the all-clear—start easy. Follow the example of the graded exercise programs offered to heart-attack victims. A typical program consists of walking, jogging and light calisthenics for forty-five minutes, three times a week. There are fifteen levels of difficulty. All participants start at Level 1, which is merely walking and light stretching. For heart-attack victims, progress to the next level depends on reduction of symptoms, absence of abnormalities in their electrocardiogram and reduction of resting pulse rate. Dr. Willem Erkelens and his colleagues at the University of Washington School of Medicine found that patients had been using such a program for as long as *nine years* without suffering another heart attack. The protective effects of the exercise were confirmed by beneficial changes in cardiovascular physiology.[103]

Exercise even combats atherosclerosis. Dr. Tom Bassler of Centinella Hospital, Inglewood, California, has shown repeatedly that jogging causes atherosclerotic plaques to disappear from the arteries.[104] The mechanisms are not yet understood, but probably involve a scouring action of the raised level of high-density lipoproteins caused by exercise and the dissolving of cholesterol and mineral deposits on the arterial walls. Atherosclerosis is one of the main ways in which the human body ages, so reversal of this disease can truly be called rejuvenation. In combination with optimum nutrition, we will soon be seeing the effects of jogging in wise individuals throughout America. They are fast becoming the youngest "oldsters" in history. Join us. I have more than a suspicion that a superhealthy heart is a happy one too.

CHAPTER 10

YOU CAN PREVENT CANCER

TODAY ONE AMERICAN in every five dies of cancer.[1] The latest figures (1982) show that of forty-two countries, twenty-five are better than America at preventing cancer in men, and twenty-three in women. We might expect countries with equivalent medicine and less pollution, like Australia, Canada and Japan, to be superior. But now countries like Greece, Paraguay, Spain, Thailand, Chile and Venezuela have far less cancer than America. With our technology the cancer record is a tragedy.

The National Cancer Institute puts the total new cancers for 1982 at 835,000.[2] Table 10 shows the twelve worst cancer killers in order of their death-dealing potential. For common cancers of the colon, rectum, ovaries, mouth and bladder and for leukemia, the chances of surviving five years after they are discovered are less than fifty-fifty. The chances of being in optimum health ever again are very small indeed. For the common cancers of the lung, liver, pancreas, stomach and brain, the chances of survival are minute. For all cancers together, the chance of surviving five years is 41 percent for whites and 32 percent for blacks. The overall improvement since 1960 is only 2 percent and 3 percent respectively. With these figures there is little merit in attempting to discuss *advances* in cancer treatment.

Table 10: New Cancer Cases and Cancer Death 1982 (The twelve worst cancer killers in order of the number of deaths they cause)

	Your Chance of Surviving Five Years			New Cases 1982
		WHITE	BLACK	
Lung		10%	7%	129,000
Liver		Not given: very small		13,100
Pancreas		Not given: almost nil		24,800
Stomach		13%	13%	24,200
Brain		20%	19%	12,400
Ovary		36%	32%	18,000
Leukemia	Acute	28%	No figures available	
	Chronic	51%	No figures available	23,500
Mouth		44%	No figures available	26,800
Colon and Rectum		48%	35%	123,000
Bladder		61%	34%	37,100
Breast		68%	51%	112,900

Medicine Does Not Prevent Cancer

In breast cancer we do see an improvement—or do we? In 1963 there were sixty-four thousand cases of breast cancer in women of all ages. The National Cancer Institute puts new cases at 112,900 for 1982. In 1963 the *five-year survival rate* for breast cancer, which political fudging sometimes calls a *cure,* was 53 percent for white women and 46 percent for black women. Despite the billions of dollars gulped by research, the survival rates today have improved by only 5 percent. In the early 1960's twenty-five thousand American women were dying each year of breast cancer; now thirty-seven thousand are dying each year.[3] Unfortunately, the number of cases of breast cancer has increased much faster than the ability of medicine to treat it.

Since 1960, when the billion-dollar ball of cancer research really started rolling, applied medicine has made very little improvement. Advances have been made in treatment of some rare forms of cancer. The chance of five-year survival for Hodgkin's disease, for example, has risen from 40 percent to 67 percent. For some forms of leukemia it has risen from 5 percent to 26 percent. But the total number of cases of Hodgkin's estimated for 1982 is seven thousand. For the successfully treatable leukemias, the figure is about eighty-five hundred.[4] The advances are good news for those who get these rare cancers. But compared with the 129,000 new cases of lung cancer, of which 119,000 will die of the disease, they are drops in the bucket.

For cancers of the brain, esophagus, lung and liver, the five-year survival rate has improved by only 1 percent to 2 percent in the last twenty years. And most of this improvement can be attributed to better prevention of complications and infections resulting from the cancer treatment. For other cancers, such as the 24,200 new cases of stomach cancer in 1982, the 26,800 new cases of mouth cancer and the 18,000 new cases of ovary cancer, the very low "cure" rates have hardly changed at all since 1960.

The increasing numbers of incurable cancer cases are only one side of the problem. Our food and environmental pollution is spreading the cancer net. Cancer used to be thought of as a disease of old age. Today it is appearing in people who are younger and younger. Cancer is now the leading disease killer in young adults aged fifteen to thirty-five, the time when they should be enjoying their most vital health. For young men leukemia has become the worst killer. For young women it is breast cancer. In fact, cancer is now *the leading cause of death* of American women from age fifteen to fifty-five, beating cardiovascular disease, accidents, liver disease, diabetes, suicide, homicide and all other causes.[5]

Early Detection Helps—Sometimes

Pap smears work. Each time I go into Cornell University Library, the wise old bronze face of George Papanicolaou merits a nod of respect for his patient work in developing the test that gives women a better chance of survival by early detection of cervical cancer. Breast self-examination has some utility also, and proctoscopy and colonoscopy for discovery of early colon and rectal cancer increase survival rates. But most detective medicine aimed at early discovery of cancer is unsuccessful.[6] For the most common cancer—of the lung—in 1979 the Surgeon General concluded that "early identification techniques such as chest X rays and sputum examination generally do not discover lung cancer before it has spread."[7]

Even early detection of breast and cervical cancers is now in question. Many diagnosed cancers are not clinically evident. They show no lumps, growths or symptoms. They are confirmed only by biopsy findings of small numbers of cancerous cells. This used to be considered a definitive sign. Now, in February 1982, Dr. Robert Hutter, president of the American Cancer Society, has raised serious doubts that many of these cancers would have developed into a life-threatening disease at all, *whether they were treated or not.* The question now is whether many of the "cured" early cancers are really cancers.[8] If not, then the cure rates are even worse than we thought, because they have been inflated by a lot of healthy people being "successfully" treated for imaginary diseases.

We cannot blame physicians for trying to catch cancer early. The disease develops silently for years inside you. When it finally shows, in most cases the body is too degenerated for even the best of treatments. The only answer is prevention. Medicine cannot help you prevent cancer. Prevention is the personal responsibility of every individual. Fortunately, recent advances in science can help you.

We Know What Causes Cancer

It is hard to imagine that substances which do not make you ill immediately can possibly cause such a serious disease as cancer. It is even harder to accept that the government would not immediately ban their use, once they had been shown to cause cancer. Yet we know now that most cancers are caused by exposure to what used to be thought of as harmless substances. Remember, soldiers who were concerned about Agent Orange when they saw the devastation it caused to plant life were treated to demonstrations of officers *drinking* a glass of it to prove it was safe. We know now just how "safe" it is.

Most cancers are caused by the effects of airborne carcinogens like asbestos, vinyl chlorides, lead, herbicides and tobacco smoke on the nose, mouth, throat and lungs, by the effects of foodborne carcinogens like aflatoxin, pesticide residues and nitrosamines on the stomach and intestines, and by the effects of carcinogens carried in body wastes to the walls of the bladder and colon.[9]

You are a hollow tube. From mouth to rectum is one continuous tunnel. The lungs, a side chamber off the tunnel, are particularly vulnerable, because their delicate tissues come into contact with the air and anything carried by it. The nose, another entry point, is important because it gives access to the underside of the brain, through a thin shield of tissue called the olfactory epithelium. By eating, drinking and breathing, the tunnel is brought into direct contact with the external environment and the carcinogens it contains. It is through this contact that the vast majority of cancers occur.

In 1979 the Surgeon General reported that twenty-three hundred different chemicals are now suspected carcinogens.[10] Your occupation, lifestyle and dietary habits determine to a large extent how much you come into contact with them. Once the degree of contact surpasses your body defenses, the seed of cancer is planted. Medicine cannot help you avoid it. You must help yourself. The precautions necessary to prevent cancer are not difficult or restrictive. They are no more arduous than cleaning your teeth. If you do that every day to prevent the minor affliction of cavities, then you should be far more motivated to prevent death by cancer.

I Would Rather Have Medflies Than Cancer

Pesticides are potent carcinogens. So are many industrial chemicals. We can no longer avoid them all, because they have invaded our water, soils, vegetables and meats. If you grow vegetables, or even lawns, use pesticides and herbicides as little as possible—and carefully. It amazes me to see how people will protect their hands with gloves from many agricultural chemicals, while gagging on the smells. The same applies to household chemicals. Women especially go to great lengths to protect their hands from bleaches, oven cleaners and insect sprays, while neglecting entirely the much more delicate tissues of the nose, throat and lungs. Use a mask. Many cancers start from breathing in carcinogens. We have a strict rule around the laboratory. What it amounts to is: If you can't eat it, don't sniff it.

Table 11 shows some common pesticides and other industrial chemicals that have been reported by the World Health Organization, the International Agency for Research on Cancer or the National Cancer Institute to cause cancer in humans or at least in one other mammal.[11] Some carcinogens are long known. Others have been indicted only recently. The public is well versed in the cancer dangers of asbestos. But innocent-looking plastics can pose equal dangers. Every form of contact with them should be avoided. For example, keep yourself and your children away from urea formaldehyde foam, used extensively for packing padding and insulating. Warn your offspring of the dangers of chewing plastics, PVC clothing or anything containing them. If you are one of the unfortunate people who bought a house or trailer insulated with urea foam, have yourself and your family examined immediately by a cancer specialist familiar with the urea formaldehyde studies, and competently trained in nutrition. If there are any positive tests, get the best lawyer you can. With thousands of people likely to be affected in the next ten years, industry will be putting up a big flak screen.

Table 11: Carcinogenic Pesticides and Chemicals in Common Use (Shown to cause cancer in man or at least one mammal species)

Substance	*Form of Cancer*
Amitrole	Thyroid, Liver
Aramite	Liver
Arsenic compounds	Skin, Lung
Asbestos	Lung
Carbon tetrachloride	Liver
Chloroform	Liver, Kidney
DDT and similar compounds	Liver
Dibromo-3-chloropropane	Stomach
Dieldrin	Liver
Ethylene dibromide	Stomach
Formaldehyde	Mucous membranes
Lead salts	Kidney
Lindane	Liver
Monuron	Liver
Polychlorinated biphenyls (PCBs)	Liver
Propiolactone	Skin
Terpene polychlorinates	Liver
Trichloroethylene	Liver
Vinyl chloride	Lung, Liver, Brain

See references 16, 20, 21.

As a result of exposure to vinyl chlorides, workers in the vinyl plastics industries have double the risk of lung cancer, a four times greater risk of brain cancer and a *two hundred times* greater risk of liver cancer than the general population.[12] The chances of surviving liver cancer are virtually nil.[13] These are very good reasons for continual monitoring of the air by a siren-attached system in these industries, and for avoiding living on their downwind side.

If you want to prevent cancer, it is sensible to avoid all industrial and household chemicals. Especially avoid breathing them into your body. Before there is sufficient evidence to get regulations made to restrict their use, many thousands of people must suffer. Don't be one of them. As the Surgeon General warns, in America new compounds are being introduced continually at the rate of over one thousand a year, "and health problems caused by some compounds in use today may not be known until the twenty-first century."[14] If that sounds unbelievable, remember that it was not until 1975 that the FDA prohibited the use of vinyl chloride in making plastic food containers,[15] although the evidence condemning it as a carcinogen had been accumulating for twenty years.

Where There's Smoke, There's Cancer

We have already discussed the effects of smoking in depleting the body of nutrients, damaging the immune system and slowly destroying the cardiovascular system. Smoking's worst effect, however, is cancer. The Surgeon General emphasizes that more than 80 percent of lung cancers and up to 50 percent of bladder cancers would be prevented if people stopped smoking.[16] The chance of surviving bladder cancer is less than fifty-fifty. With lung cancer it is still *less than 10 percent.*

Each five days of moderate smoking reduces your lifespan by one day. You give up seventy days of life a year. Every five smoking years your potential lifespan is reduced by one. There is no safe level of smoking. Being a so-called noninhaler doesn't help either. A long study begun in 1959 has shown recently that forty-five to fifty-five-year-old male smokers who were "noninhalers" had a 40 percent higher mortality rate than nonsmokers.[17]

By 1980 male deaths from lung cancer, attributable mainly to smoking, had increased sevenfold since 1940, despite all the warnings, the smoking controls, the filter cigarettes, the low-tar, low-nicotine brands. For women there has been an abrupt threefold increase in lung cancer since 1960. Over thirty-one thousand American women will die of it in 1982. And the National Cancer Institute predicts they will be replaced by another thirty eight thousand new cases.[18] What a powerful drug nicotine is, that people will take such risks for its pleasures!

The latest assessments by the Surgeon General and by other independent scientists show that attempts to make a "safe" cigarette have been a total failure.[19] This is not surprising. Apart from nicotine tars and carbon monoxide, literally hundreds of other chemicals are added to tobacco. So far, the Food and Drug Administration has avoided taking on the huge tobacco lobby to force manufacturers to disclose what particular chemicals they are using. Only you, the public, can make them do so. Even if you are not a smoker, there is now reliable evidence that other people smoking near you expose you to respiratory, cardiovascular and carcinogenic effects of smoking.[20] Amazing how social crimes linger. We wouldn't let anyone spray us with Agent Orange. It is time smokers paid handsomely for the privilege of permission to cause cancer in others.

Medication Can Cause Cancer

Many, many drugs are carcinogenic, from the once-common analgesic phenacetin to the synthetic hormone diethylstilbestrol (DES).[21] The 1,470 pages of the *American Medical Association Drug Evaluations* handbook read like a horror story.[22] Space makes it impossible even to list the cancer suspects here. Five minutes with this volume is sufficient to convince anyone that drugs should be used only for the really ill.

Everything from contraceptive pills to the common antibiotics are suspected of causing human cancer.[23] As a side effect, some of the anticancer drugs *cause* cancer, the disease they are meant to correct. There is now considerable action being taken throughout the medical community to protect physicians, nurses and laboratory staff from contracting cancer as a result of handling these drugs.

Further, the procedures most used to treat cancer—surgery, chemotherapy and radiation therapy—themselves *cause* new cancers. In books *by* physicians *for* physicians, there are multiple instances of tumor-causing treatment procedures.[24] I cannot say why this evidence has not received more public attention. But in October 1981 the National Cancer Institute was called before congressional hearings where it was accused of gross mismanagement of the cancer program by legislators and by the Food and Drug Administration. The investigation is proceeding.[25]

Another medical risk for cancer is X rays. They used to be thought so harmless and used so freely that in the 1950's machines were common in shoe shops in Britain and America, using X rays to see if you had a good shoe-fitting. Even now, it is commonplace for Americans to have at least one routine X ray every year. Yet world authority on radiation damage Dr. John Gofman, professor of medical physics at the University of California, has shown conclusively that repeated chest X rays cause breast cancer and increase the risk of leukemia in women.[26] For men, those who receive more than twenty X rays anywhere from chest to navel *double* their risk of leukemia. More than forty such X rays increases the risk of leukemia by *seven times*.[27] Now, a lot of physicians, like distinguished pediatrician Dr. Robert Mendelsohn of the University of Illinois, believe that any X ray is hazardous to your health.[28] Do not have X rays unless they are essential to prescribed medical treatment. X rays for insurance purposes, job applications and cosmetic dentistry are dangerous misapplications of medicine.

All the more powerful drugs and medical procedures are by prescription only, so it is your physician's responsibility to protect you against their unwanted effects. Many people, however, consistently misuse prescribed medication. It is foolish, not only for the risk of cancer, but also for all the other degenerative diseases that are documented side effects of many prescription drugs.[29] The answer is clear. Use prescribed drugs only in dire necessity, and only after you have had the risks and side effects fully explained. Limit your over-the-counter medication to occasional aspirin. And for any other medical procedure, ask your physician straight, no-nonsense questions regarding necessity and risk. If he refuses or fails to answer them, get another physician—one competently trained in nutrition. The Huxley Institute in New York City can give you the name of such a physician in your area.

Even Food Can Cause Cancer

If you are serious about preventing cancer, then realize that many carcinogens have been identified recently that occur *naturally* in food or as a result of storage, processing or cooking. We will examine some important ones. Psoralens, found in all parsnips, are powerful carcinogens. Recent studies from a number of laboratories show that they cause cancer readily in animals.[30] We can only guess at the number of cases of human cancer to which parsnips have contributed. Do not eat them.

Unsaturated fats that have been heated, such as margarine and all cooking oils (except cold-pressed oils), have lost their antioxidants and are very prone to oxidation. The oxidation reaction produces many carcinogens, such as hydroperoxides, aldehydes and expoxides. So use only cold-pressed cooking oils. Never use any oil, margarine or vegetable shortening that has a hint of rancidity. The common practice of "saving" cooking fats that have already been used should be abandoned.

We have already examined how nitrates in foods produce carcinogenic nitrosamines in storage, in cooking and in the stomach. Preserved and tinned meats and preserved sausages, or any meat product containing nitrates or nitrites, should be avoided. Hamburger and processed meats often have these substances added, especially where they are stored in bulk. Fast-food franchises and restaurant chains are likely suspects.

Aflatoxin Kills

Don't eat nuts or seeds that have the least suspicion of moldiness or rancidity. The molds produce potent carcinogens called aflatoxins. Discard all cheese that has gone moldy also. It may contain a carcinogen called sterigmatocystin as well as aflatoxin. Unfortunately for gourmets, this warning includes all deliberately molded cheeses, such as gorgonzola and blue cheese. It is difficult to accept that eating such traditional foods contributes to cancer. On hearing me present the data on cheese carcinogens, one colleague exclaimed, "Hell! Another of my favorite vices is carcinogenic. Why wasn't I born in the nineteenth century, when we knew nothing about it?" It is not *that* restrictive to prevent cancer. Remember, it is continual abuse, the regular drip-drip of poisons, which overcomes the body's defenses. Occasionally enjoying a humming cheese is not going to hurt you.

We didn't realize the dangers of aflatoxin until the 1960's, when millions of poultry died in Britain as a result of eating moldy peanuts imported from South America.[31] Then, millions of trout in California trout farms died of liver cancer, also from aflatoxin. The carcinogen responsible, aflatoxin, eluded identification for nearly two years. Now, we know that aflatoxin develops in fungi that grow on cereals, seeds and nuts during storage without proper heat, moisture and humidity controls. In monkeys aflatoxin takes about six years to produce liver cancer—but it does so inevitably.[32]

Our exposure to this carcinogen has been increasing rapidly alongside the growth of modern methods of long-term food storage. Since 1970 all developed countries have established aflatoxin controls, but they vary widely. Monitoring is very difficult.[33] Harvesting, storage and distribution methods that were developed to suit space-age technology have had to be radically changed. Costs are huge, and likely to be avoided as far as possible by industry.

There is little hope of controlling the storage of foods that originate outside the United States. Your safeguards are wise shopping and wise use of the detectors of your own body. Buy only grains, seeds and nuts you know are fresh. Locally grown, small-volume products are therefore preferable. Even with these, use the sensitive receptors of your eyes, nose and mouth to detect bitterness, moldiness, discoloration or "old" appearance of foods. Don't buy them if you find any signs, and discard the foods if you find signs at home. Most packaged, shelled nuts, for example, are far too deteriorated to be safe. You cannot solve the problem by scrubbing, peeling or cooking either. Some of the aflatoxins in livestock feed survive all the processes of animal digestion, plus the stringent procedures of pasteurization and homogenization, and appear intact and biologically active in commercial milk.

Coffee is Probably Carcinogenic

Coffee is now implicated in cancer of the pancreas.[34] In 1981 Dr. Brian MacMahon and his colleagues at Harvard found that heavy coffee drinking was the only variable that separated 369 pancreatic cancer patients from 644 other patients. More than five cups a day brings a three times greater risk of cancer than no coffee at all. Supporting evidence comes from studies of Mormons and Seventh Day Adventists. They don't drink coffee and very rarely get pancreatic cancer. In two couples among the cancer patients in Dr. MacMahon's study, both husband and wife had pancreatic cancer. Both were heavy coffee drinkers. The probability of husband and wife getting the same cancer by unconnected coincidence is very small. While this evidence is not conclusive, it confirms many scattered reports over the last twenty years.

Coffee contains many biologically active substances. One of its enzymes, called galactosidase, for example, is strong enough to destroy the antigens which protect your particular blood type.

It will readily change type B blood into type O. So decaffeinated coffee is not a safe switch as far as cancer is concerned. The carcinogen in coffee is unlikely to be caffeine. There is no association of heavy tea drinking with cancer, and tea has nearly as much of caffeinelike chemicals as coffee. So, reduce the coffee habit. Cancer of the pancreas may take twenty years to show. Once it does, chances of survival are almost nil.[35]

Three other common sources of food carcinogens are burning and charring of protein during cooking, red wine and tap water. The hazards of water are covered in Chapter 12. In France red wine has been reliably associated with stomach cancer. The carcinogens may be in the grapes (a substance called guercetin is one), or may result from added chemicals or processes used in the manufacture of wine. It is gratifying to see the recent shift to white wines in America. Charring of protein foods such as meat and cheese is a recently discovered cancer hazard. The evidence is still being evaluated. Meanwhile, it is easy insurance to cut off the burned bits. If you think I am exaggerating the dangers, then know that in February 1982 the National Cancer Advisory Board gave top priority to research on food carcinogens, including all those discussed above. They suggested that carcinogens which develop in food may turn out to be more important in the development of cancer than all the industrial chemicals put together.[36]

The Cancer Prevention Lifestyle

Obesity causes cancer. In 1959 the American Cancer Society started a twenty-year study of more than one million Americans spread over twenty-five different states to find out what life conditions correlate with cancer. A massive and representative study. They found that men who are more than 40 percent overweight have higher rates of cancer of the colon, rectum and prostate gland. Women who are 40 percent or more overweight have higher rates of cancer of the ovaries, uterus, gall bladder and breast.[37] The evidence is clear. The preventive strategy against obesity is detailed in Chapter 8. Being slim is an anticancer decision.

Being very slim may be better still. In Chapter 4 we discussed the overall anti-aging effect of eating small. A major component of this effect may be the prevention of kinds of degeneration that produce cancer. Underfeeding studies with animals show lower rates of all kinds of cancer. The latest one, done at the University of California Medical School by world-renowned gerontologist Dr. Roy Walford and his colleagues, showed that mice given small meals, but meals enriched with vitamins and minerals, had far less cancer and lived 10 percent to 20 percent longer than control mice given free access to normal chow.[38] The important advance in this study is that the underfeeding was not started until the mice were nearly middle-aged. So, there is hope for all of us.

Fiber Protects, Fats Kill

The type of diet eaten is important also. A recent comparison of dietary patterns and incidence of colon and rectum cancer in twenty countries has shown definite associations.[39] High-fat, low-fiber diets, the usual American pattern, show very high rates of colon and rectal cancer. Conversely, low-fat, high-fiber diets show a very low rate. Argentina and Uruguay which, like America, eat a lot of beef (high in fat), have huge rates of colon and rectal cancer compared with the low rates of neighboring South American countries.[40] Japan has a very low-fat diet—and very low rates of colon and rectal cancer. But in Japanese who migrate to America and adopt American food, the rates jump by 700 percent![41]

Probably the cancer develops from three interrelated sources. First, the body expels many carcinogens in feces. Second, high-fat diets result in increased bile acids in the bowel.[42] Bacteria act on these to produce carcinogens or cocarcinogens which enable carcinogenic substances in food wastes to attack the bowel walls. Third, low-fiber diets reduce the water in the bowel, resulting in a greater concentration of injurious bile acids. They also delay the passage of feces, giving a longer time of contact between the carcinogens and the bowel. In America average passage time from mouth to elimination is forty-eight to seventy-two hours. On high-fiber diets it is twenty-four to thirty-six hours.[43]

Colon and rectal cancers are now the second most common cancers in America, with 123,000 new cases in 1982. There is little doubt this dreadful disease is almost entirely preventable by a simple change of diet. It is the most important reason why red meats should figure lightly, if at all, in your food. Instead, make whole grain breads and cereals, raw fruits and vegetables the bulk of your daily diet.

High-fat diets are also involved in breast cancer. Comparisons between numerous countries have shown that the higher the level of fats in the diet, the higher the rate of breast cancer.[44] Like many cancers, the "seed" is most likely to be planted *many years before,* during puberty, during the development of the breasts. Probably the fats interfere with hormonal cycles, and puberty is a very vulnerable period. Japan has a very low-fat diet and about one sixth the breast cancer of America. Adult Japanese women who migrate to America and adopt the American diet remain at fairly low risk, but their young daughters, raised here, get breast cancer in adulthood at about the same rate as Americans.[45] Even if you will not avoid fats, it is a tragedy to teach the meat-gorging habit to your daughters.

Switching to unsaturated fats will not help you. We have already discussed the dangers of cooking oils and margarines which have lost their natural antioxidants during processing. They oxidize rapidly in storage, cooking and inside you, to produce myriads of our old enemies the free radicals, which can damage any body function easily. Polyunsaturated fats, low in cholesterol and widely touted as being safer than animal fats, cause *more* cancer in experimental animals than saturated fats.[46]

These studies prompted scientists to see what had happened to all those people in the 1960's who were put on unsaturated fats/low-cholesterol diets to control their cholesterol levels, and supposedly prevent cardiovascular disease. The unfortunate results show how much more careful medical science must be when attempting to play God with nature. In one long study, patients were given four times the usual level of unsaturated fats in their diets and half the usual level of cholesterol. There is little evidence that the manipulation helped cardiovascular disease. What did occur was increased rates of various kinds of fatal cancers.[47] Two reexaminations of the human studies on unsaturated fats and cardiovascular disease show little evidence of increased cancer.[48] But there is some doubt that the patients stuck to the diets. The cancer-producing effects of polyunsaturated fats in human patients have now been confirmed.[49]

We continue to be bludgeoned with advertisements to use unsaturated fats for two reasons. First, the variety of our diets is supposed to protect us by providing the necessary antioxidants. But we know from previous chapters that most American diets are sadly deficient in these life-preserving substances. Second, when the evils of saturated fats were discovered in the 1960's, the food industry made a very costly switch to vegetable fats. Now, billions of dollars are invested in the unsaturated fats, and advertising does a good job of selling them. As we discussed in Chapter 9, they do no good for cardiovascular disease. And the evidence here indicates that they *increase* the risk of cancer. The prevention lifestyle rule is: Avoid fats of all kinds.

Vitamins Prevent Cancer

We have known for many years that Vitamin A deficiency increases the risk of cancer enormously.[50] The scientific debate has been: How much Vitamin A is best? In 1976 and 1977 Dr. Michael Sporn of the National Cancer Institute showed that high supplemental Vitamin A prevents cancer in experimental animals exposed to carcinogenic chemicals.[51] It is highly successful in preventing cancer of the skin, windpipe, bronchial tubes, breast, stomach, bladder, cervix and vagina.

You are not in an experiment, but you are a human animal exposed to carcinogenic chemicals. Even if you follow all the advice in this book, every day you ingest at least one hundred manufactured chemicals known to be carcinogenic. So it is sensible never to let your Vitamin A store get low. Eat foods rich in this vitamin, such as carrots, unsulphured dried apricots, parsley, broccoli, green onions, romaine lettuce and nectarines. Also, follow the instructions in Chapter 6 to work out your daily supplement.

In 1981 a nineteen-year study of 1,950 men showed that high intake of Provitamin A, the form of Vitamin A found in carrots, is protective against lung cancer, *even among smokers.*[52] These extremely important findings have led to many people trying to obtain synthetic Vitamin A, which is less toxic in large amounts than the usual supplement, retinol. Two of these synthetics are cis retinoic acid and beta-carotene. Both are now available commercially from Hoffman La Roche. But you are far better off eating carrots regularly. You don't have to do it every day, because Vitamin A is stored in the human body.

The involvement of B vitamins in cancer is complex and still poorly understood. Deficiency of folic acid, very common in America, reduces the resistance of experimental animals to cancer of the trachea and colon.[53] Deficiencies of Vitamin B_{12} and choline are also involved. Supplements of Vitamin B_2 inhibit development of liver cancer in rats.[54] Remember that the whole B complex only works synergistically. No studies have yet been done to show how this basic physiological function occurs. Until such studies are done, we do not know how much protection against cancer is afforded by the B vitamins.

We do know about Vitamin C. It does protect us against cancer.[55] Thanks to Dr. Linus Pauling's sticking to his guns over many years against enormous criticism, other investigators have been stimulated to examine the effects of this deceptively simple substance. We have already discussed how it maintains immune function. An immune function disorder is part of most cancers. I am currently engaged in studies which I hope will show that Vitamin C protects immune function directly during disease. Dr. Robert Yonemoto, director of the Cancer Department of City of Hope National Medical Center in California, has already published important findings that Vitamin C improves immune function in patients undergoing conventional therapy for breast cancer.[56]

Vitamin C has many other actions in the body, however, an important one being its antioxidant activity. Whatever the mechanism, it inhibits cancer reliably in experimental animals.[57] It also confers resistance to the progress of cancer even after it is established in the body. Patients supplemented with Vitamin C have a death rate from cancer between 40 percent and 60 percent less than those on "normal" diets. This decrease in death rate gives an increased lifespan of eight to eleven years.[58] It is a happy outcome of the Vitamin C controversy that Dr. Pauling has at last convinced the National Cancer Institute of the vitamin's benefits. Now hale and hearty, having outlived his major critics, he continues to pursue his research under grants from this august body.

One other vitamin has known effects on cancer. Vitamin E is important because of its antioxidant activity, especially in the protection of cell membranes. Along with Vitamin C and selenium, it may also be important in protecting the intestines and colon, as some of it fails to be digested and passes through the body with food wastes. As Vitamin E is fat-soluble, it retards putrefaction of fecal fat. The colon walls are therefore subjected to less potential injury. In fact, there is considerable evidence that the human organism evolved to eat large quantities of Vitamins C and E daily.[59] Part of the natural function of these nutrients in the human body is to pass through it along with food residues to directly protect the bowels (and the bladder) from injurious effects of the body's own wastes during the process of their elimination. Consequently, vitamins excreted in your urine and feces may not be the indication of unwise oversupplementation that they are commonly taken for. They may well be an essential component of the body's own protective wisdom.

Little is known about interactions between carcinogens and the remainder of the vitamins and essential minerals. Deficiency of the mineral iodine, very common in America, is associated with increased thyroid cancer in experimental animals.[60] Magnesium deficiency is also involved in cancer. However, the only mineral with clear anticancer effects is selenium. Recently, carefully controlled studies by Dr. Maryce Jacobs of the University of Nebraska and Dr. Clark Griffin of the University of Texas have confirmed earlier studies that dietary selenium supplementation can prevent some cancers in experimental animals exposed to powerful chemical carcinogens. This protection has been confirmed for colon, liver and lung carcinogens.[61]

The antioxidant action of selenium is one mechanism involved. But it is not the only one. Selenium will protect animals even from injections of actual living cancers, grown for the purpose in the laboratory. Without the supplemental selenium these cultured cancers "take" readily and produce cancer in the animals. Also, if selenium is added to the cancer cultures, no cancers appear when they are subsequently injected into animals, even if the animals themselves are not receiving selenium supplements.[62]

So, selenium must have a variety of inhibiting effects on cancer. For prevention of cancer, Dr. Gerhard Schrauzer has shown that selenium in the drinking water of animals reduces the risk of breast cancer substantially.[63] Epidemiological studies of human cancer show that in areas where selenium is low in the soil and water, there is increased incidence of breast and colon or rectal cancer.[64] As we have seen in earlier chapters, selenium is deficient in the diet of most Americans. If you want to prevent cancer, you will follow the directions given in Chapters 6 and 7 to ensure it is not deficient in yours.

The mass of findings about nutrient effects against cancer is surprising. All these strong preventive effects have been found with single nutrients, yet we know that nutrients can operate only by multiple interactions with each other. All these studies have been relying on the diet to provide the missing nutrient links. Not one investigator has tested the effects of a complete vitamin and mineral supplement. Yet all the evidence in this book points to complete supplementation being far more effective than single nutrients in preventing degenerative disease. The simple procedure of daily use of an individually designed supplement, in conjunction with a good diet, will do far more to reduce cancer in America than all the efforts, past and future, of physicians, clinics and hospitals combined.

In sharp contrast to even ten years ago, many medical scientists now share this belief. In 1977 eminent British cancer specialist Sir Richard Doll echoed the feeling of many of us when he said, "I have laid particular stress on diet because I suspect that in the next few years the main advances in our knowledge of how to control cancer will come from studying this aspect of our environment."[65]

Do not fear cancer. I remember Dr. Lewis Thomas, president of the prestigious Sloan-Kettering Cancer Hospital in New York, emphasizing the terrible public dread of this disease. He commented that the public belief today "seems to be that the body is fundamentally flawed."[66] On the contrary, as Dr. Thomas attests, the human system is incredibly tough. Daily it resists bacteria, viruses, poisons and carcinogens with ease. Give it optimum nutrition and it will repay you handsomely.

CHAPTER 11

YOU CAN PREVENT DIABETES

SUGAR DIABETES AFFLICTS more than ten million Americans. Probably twice that number are prediabetic. Their bodies have become so deficient at dealing with carbohydrates (starches and sugars) that they get recurrent incidents of hyperglycemia (high blood sugar) or hypoglycemia (low blood sugar). They suffer incessant hunger and thirst, weakness, tremor, nausea, giddiness, anxiety or irritability. They risk overt diabetes every day. By careless or ignorant nutrition habits, another twenty million are "training" themselves to develop these conditions. The mechanisms that maintain their blood sugar at a stable level have been abused to the brink of disorder. They cannot go more than four hours or so without feeling the need for a pick-me-up snack. Although some diabetes results from genetic defects, viral infections and organ damage,[1] many cases follow the above route. *Almost all that do are preventable.*

At my clinic we examined thirty apparently healthy students between the ages of eighteen and twenty-five to see if we could find any evidence of disturbed carbohydrate metabolism. At these ages we expected three cases at most from a sample of this size. To our great surprise, following a mere five-and-a-half-hour fast, nine young women and seven young men reported at least one symptom. Twelve of these students also showed tremor, evidence of giddiness, irritability or abnormally low blood sugar. All reported a usual dietary pattern of snacking every two to three hours during the day, often on processed carbohydrate and little else. Nine were completely unaware that they had developed this dependence on empty calories.

Our sample was tiny, but our findings agree with those of numerous other studies that the seed of adult-onset diabetes is probably planted very early in adult life. Worse, we know now that in many cases of mild disturbance of sugar metabolism, such as we found in our student sample, the degeneration of eyes, kidneys and blood vessels that typically shows in diabetes *is already taking place.*[2] We know also that this degeneration can be reversed if caught early enough.[3] But if people do not even suspect it is happening . . .

These findings help explain why, for the last thirty years, America has had one of the highest rates of diabetic death and complications in the world. We have almost five times the rate of Japan, twice the rate of Britain and a higher rate than fifteen other developed countries. Despite our massive medical effort against diabetes, the incidence of this fearsome degenerative disease is steadily increasing.[4] So much so that overseas researchers now call it the "American candy syndrome."

The Insulin Myths

It is still a popular belief that diabetes develops because the body gradually loses its ability to produce insulin, the hormone made by the pancreas gland that regulates the body's use of sugar. Some unfortunate people do have this problem, but many diabetics produce just as much insulin, just as rapidly, as nondiabetics.[5] The prediabetic condition, which we are concerned to prevent from progressing into diabetes, often shows *high* blood insulin.[6] The ability to produce insulin may be perfectly normal. But for a variety of reasons it fails to control blood sugar. The most common fault is a loss of sensitivity in the cells that recognize the level of sugar in the blood and enable insulin to react with it.[7] So sugar and insulin continue to circulate in the bloodstream, ignoring each other. The sugar level rises until the blood can no longer contain the excess, resulting in the typical spillover into the urine that used to be the hallmark of diabetes mellitus (the sweet urine disease).

Initially, prediabetics may notice only that they always seem to be hungry and thirsty. Then, unaccountable weakness starts to appear. Unless controlled by insulin injections, the disorder progresses insidiously to sudden coma and death. Or worse, progressive destruction of the eyes, the kidneys and the small blood vessels, resulting in blindness, gangrene, progressive amputation surgery and a lingering illness that often concludes with a fatal heart attack.

Even if insulin is used to "control" the disease, it continues to progress.[8] The lifespan and health of a "controlled" diabetic is way below average. In a typical study completed in 1978, Drs. Torsten Deckert and Morgens Larsen at the Steno Memorial Hospital in Copenhagen charted the lives of 800 diabetic men and 650 diabetic women. All had previously developed diabetes before age thirty-one. All but thirteen were "controlled" with insulin. Deckert and Larsen matched the diabetic patients with same-age healthy men and women in the normal population of Denmark. As the disease progressed, nearly all the patients developed serious degenerative complications. By 1976 only 40 percent of them were still alive, compared with 90 percent of the control population.[9] Fortunately, nutrition can do a lot to prevent your becoming a similar statistic of this sickness.

Fats Can Cause Diabetes

The usual prediabetic, a person whose body is losing its ability to deal with sugar (and other carbohydrates), shows *high* blood sugar, *high* blood insulin and *high* blood fats (triglycerides).[10] And studies of confirmed diabetics show that high levels of blood fats interfere with the ability of the body to use insulin.[11] We know blood fats are major culprits, because if we lower them, the body's use of insulin returns to normal.[12]

Lowering blood fats (triglycerides) is not so easy, because the very loss of interaction between insulin and sugar that high triglycerides cause also serves to keep fat levels up. This is because the high level of insulin, which is inhibited from dealing with the sugar, goes to the liver, where it is used up by the body in making excess triglycerides.[13] So, it's a vicious cycle. The more triglycerides the body makes, the greater the interference with the insulin/sugar reaction. The body then makes even more insulin to compensate, which is then used to make even more triglycerides. Each day, the person runs a progressively greater risk of diabetes.

Happily, there are several ways out of the cycle. High blood fats are also correlated with diets high in fat. Populations in undeveloped countries that live on low-fat diets typically have low blood sugar, low triglycerides and virtually no diabetes. Diabetes is rare in the Bantu tribe, for example. Yet those Bantu who adopt city life, and with it the Western high-fat diet, quickly change to show rising blood fats and disturbances of carbohydrate metabolism at the same rate as Europeans.[14] Probably the best evidence comes from confirmed diabetics. There is no longer any doubt that low-fat diets improve the insulin mechanism and reduce the need for insulin medication.[15] So, as we saw with both cardiovascular disease and cancer, but for different reasons, avoiding dietary fats helps prevent diabetes.

Obesity Causes Diabetes

Dietary fat is not the only kind of fat you should worry about. The fat of overweight may be a worse danger. Bodily abuse over many years, which has led to the overweight endemic in America today, produces not only atherosclerosis, but diabetes too.

Obesity not only raises cholesterol levels,[16] it also raises triglyceride levels. This disorder of blood fats develops because fat cells themselves are resistant to the normal action of insulin as it tries to control the body's use of sugar. For every extra fat cell you develop, or latent fat cell you fill up, the body has to produce more and more excess insulin in an attempt to keep them nourished. It is not very successful, so a lot of the excess goes to the liver, which then produces excess triglycerides that add further to the insulin resistance, and the vicious cycle is off and running.[17] Eventually, the pancreas can no longer keep pace with the demand for insulin. Blood sugar rises to dangerous levels, and obesity diabetes is born.

Because of biochemical individuality, some people are more resistant to this process than others. They may have a stronger pancreas, one that is able to keep up the insulin flow. Or they may have large muscles. Such people can carry fat with less risk. Their higher ratio of muscle cells (which use insulin normally) to insulin-resistant fat cells helps to keep down the demand for insulin, one very good reason for maintaining an exercise program as you age. Nevertheless, at some point *all* obese people lose the battle. Abnormalities of sugar metabolism develop, and they live in the shadow of diabetes.[18]

Obesity prediabetes can be easily overcome as long as it is caught before irreversible kidney and blood-vessel damage occurs. If people of normal weight are force fed, they become obese and show the typical prediabetic condition. But as soon as they return to a normal diet and lose the weight, sugar metabolism also returns to normal.[19] It is the same for obese patients put on a reducing diet. Sugar metabolism improves in direct proportion to every pound of fat lost.[20] Even in confirmed obese diabetics, weight reduction substantially improves their sugar metabolism, lowers their blood insulin and lowers their blood triglycerides.[21] If you can find no other reason to stay slim, then perhaps saving your sight and your kidneys may give you an incentive.

Carbohydrates Can Cause Diabetes—or Prevent It

From Chapter 8 we know that almost all obesity results from eating excess calories. These are usually in the form of processed carbohydrates (starches and sugars), the pap to which most of our food is reduced today. Excess sugar is the biggest problem. Nearly twenty years ago Dr. William Ishmael of the University of Oklahoma Medical Center showed how dietary sugar causes prediabetic reactions by raising the level of triglycerides in the blood.[22] Populations that live on low-sugar diets, such as the Zulus, have very few diabetics. But Zulus who migrate to city life adopt the Western diet. Their sugar consumption goes up tenfold, and the rates of hyperglycemia, hypoglycemia and diabetes rise to the same level as that of Caucasian South Africans.[23]

One oft-quoted exception is the Pima Indian tribe of Arizona, who have a fairly low-sugar diet yet almost the highest rate in the world of adult-onset diabetes.[24] With an inexcusable lapse of logic, some researchers at the National Academy of Sciences have taken these facts to mean that dietary sugar and diabetes may be unconnected.[25] However, the Pima not only tend to have genetic predispositions to disorders of sugar metabolism, but the vast majority of diabetic Pima are obese. As we have seen, obesity causes diabetes, whether you eat a lot of sugar or not.

Some other health writers have tried to reduce the sugar risk by advising people to use unsweetened bread and cereal products. Seemingly, they fail to realize that processed starches are absorbed by the body almost as fast as sugar, and are immediately converted to sugar by bodily processes. People who martyr themselves with dry crackers in the mistaken belief that they are helping their sugar metabolism are not gaining a whit of value over the equivalent number of calories' worth of lip-smacking pecan pie.

Numerous studies now confirm this simple physiological process. In 1978, for example, noted authority on diabetes Dr. Gerald Reaven of the VA Hospital at Palo Alto, California, gave twenty-seven diabetics a diet containing 55 percent total carbohydrates (including 25 percent sucrose) or a diet containing 40 percent total carbohydrates (including the same 25 percent sucrose). Some patients had the 55 percent diet for the first week, then the 40 percent diet. Others were given the diets in reverse order. Results showed clearly that the 55 percent carbohydrate diet raises insulin and blood triglycerides much higher than the 40 percent carbohydrate diet,[26] although the proportion of sugar was the same in both.

So the proportion of simple sugar you eat as part of your carbohydrate is far less important than the proportion of total carbohydrates in your diet. From Dr. Reaven's and similar studies,[27] anyone with the slightest suspicion of a disturbance of sugar metabolism who just can't resist processed foods should keep total carbohydrates between 40 percent and 50 percent. If you *can* avoid processed foods, then, as we will see, the proportion of total carbohydrate is not so important.

When you eat the carbohydrate *is* important. Further studies by Dr. Reaven have confirmed the long-held notion that distributing your carbohydrate throughout the day is better than eating it mainly at one time. Prediabetic patients were given their carbohydrate in four equal small meals a day. They showed the same levels of blood sugar as normal persons used as controls. Given the same amount of carbohydrate at one sitting, however, their blood sugar rose into the danger range.[28] So, the second step of carbohydrate regulation is—distribute.

The complexity of carbohydrate is even more important. For many years confusion has reigned in dietary advice for prediabetics and even for confirmed diabetics, with some authorities claiming that low-carbohydrate, high-fat diets were best,[29] and others promoting high-carbohydrate, low-fat diets.[30] Argument rages back and forth at learned meetings reminiscent of small children shouting 'tis, 'tisn't, 'tis, 'tisn't, because both sides are right. The problem is that many studies prior to 1975 failed to measure the relative amounts of simple (usually processed) carbohydrate and complex carbohydrate.

Yet this distinction is the key variable. We saw in Chapter 9 that switching from simple to complex carbohydrates lowers blood-cholesterol levels. The question is, How do complex carbohydrates exert such protective effects on fat metabolism? The answer lies in the *fiber* that they contain.

Fiber Is the Key

When British physician Dr. Henry Trowell reported in the 1950's that diabetes is much lower in populations who live on high-fiber diets, he was ignored. When he showed successful control of diabetes with high dietary fiber, he was still ignored. Now, many studies show he is absolutely right. High fiber levels reliably reduce blood-sugar levels, reduce or eliminate sugar in the urine and reduce insulin requirements in diabetics.[31]

The best news for diabetics and prediabetics is that improvement in sugar metabolism is progressive. For example, at the University of Oxford, Dr. David Jenkins and his colleagues added twenty to twenty-five grams of guar per day to patients' diets. Guar is a legume, a complex carbohydrate grown in the United States for animal feed. You can make a biscuit of it that tastes a bit like Elmer's glue. Gastronomic "delights" aside, patients were able to reduce their insulin dosage progressively over twenty weeks, good evidence that the sticky fiber acts on the intestines in some as-yet-unknown way so as to repair damaged sugar metabolism.[32]

High-fiber diets also lower blood triglycerides in diabetics and prediabetics. This is not an artificial influence either, because such diets don't lower triglycerides in people with normal levels.[33] Fiber probably repairs faulty sugar metabolism by its complex effects on stomach and intestinal functioning. The human body evolved eating a high-fiber diet. The studies serve to confirm that the human body works properly only on the fuel it was designed for.

Once a high-fiber diet is adopted, the proportion of total carbohydrates to fats and proteins in the diet becomes unimportant. For example, in 1978 Dr. James Anderson of the University of Kentucky College of Medicine fed seventeen diabetics (six of them obese) high-carbohydrate diets (70 percent) containing high fiber (seventy to eighty grams a day). At the start of the study the patients were receiving between fourteen and twenty units of insulin a day. Insulin requirements dropped promptly and insulin was discontinued entirely for sixteen of the seventeen patients within fourteen days on the diet.[34] So, fortunately, to maintain normal sugar metabolism, you don't have to keep your diet low in *all* carbohydrates—just the processed carbohydrates.

Unfortunately, that's not the whole story. Even fiber comes in different forms. There are the sticky, soluble types like guar, the pectin in fruits, and Metamucil, which is made from the seeds of the psyllium plant. These dreadful-tasting substances are favored in diabetic diets because they cause the stomach to empty more slowly. Food is therefore absorbed from the intestines more gradually and does not release a sudden sugar load into a damaged system. Insoluble fiber foods like bran have just the opposite effect. They quicken gastric emptying, which may be excellent for regularity but will not slow down absorption.

For prevention of diabetes you don't have to go to either extreme, but you do have to know what constitutes a good fiber food. Potatoes, for example, are a nice middle-of-the-road complex carbohydrate. A fresh raw potato is high in just the sort of fiber you need. But if you bake it, a lot of the fiber breaks down, so that it becomes more like a processed carbohydrate. In prediabetics baked potato raises blood insulin and blood sugar just as high and just as rapidly as feeding them pure glucose.[35] You don't even have to bake the potato. Like numerous other tubers, its fiber also breaks down readily under long storage. So don't rely on potatoes for fiber, or on other root vegetables, unless you know when they were harvested.

Breads made from a preponderance of white flour, or so-called enriched flour are worse, no matter how crusty or chunky. In processing, the flour loses 90 percent of its fiber. The same goes for white rice. Yet whole wheat bread and real brown rice (not the dyed white variety) are excellent sources of fiber. Of all the enjoyable fiber foods, boiled brown rice shows the best effects in prediabetes.[36]

A good preventive diet for anyone overweight, or with even a hint of sugar problems, should contain about forty grams of fiber per thousand calories. That works out as 85 g (3 oz) of fiber per day on a 2,000-calorie diet. A typical day might offer whole grain cereal and fresh fruit for breakfast, mixed whole grain breads with poultry, fish or cheese and raw fruit and vegetables for lunch, and whole grain bread with poultry, seafood or eggs, cooked fresh vegetables and brown rice for dinner, with raw or cooked fresh fruit desserts. Snacks can be whole grain or brown-rice cookies, crudités or fruit. Such a diet is not only sensible for those trying to avoid diabetes, it forms an excellent basis for anyone concerned with preserving good health.

Vitamins Combat Diabetes

None of the dietary manipulations will work for long if the body lacks essential nutrients. While keeping in mind that no vitamin works alone, we will look at a few examples of substances related to the degenerative changes that precede and accompany diabetes. Riboflavin is intimately involved in sugar metabolism. Riboflavin deficiency in animals causes disorders of glucose tolerance similar to those seen in diabetics.[37] Mice made even moderately riboflavin deficient show large disturbances of blood sugar and blood insulin following a feeding of glucose. Sixty minutes after the feeding they show the typical prediabetic pattern of high blood glucose and high blood insulin, indicating a severe disorder of the mechanism whereby insulin deals with sugar in the blood. Riboflavin supplements quickly restore these responses to normal.[38]

Vitamin E is also an important preventive measure for anyone with evidence of glucose intolerance. The inevitable accompaniment of this problem is the gradual death of peripheral blood vessels. The first to go are the tiny capillaries that nourish the hands and feet, fingers and toes. There is firm evidence that supplemental Vitamin E is beneficial in maintaining peripheral circulation in a variety of vascular diseases.[39] This vitamin also helps to maintain normal levels of blood fats,[40] and thereby reduces cardiovascular risk, so is important to anyone whose signs of prediabetes show that his risk is increased.

Vitamin C is similarly important. Accelerated atherosclerosis is also an inevitable accompaniment of the progression of diabetes. As we saw in Chapter 9, Vitamin C has multiple effects on the arteries. Even in confirmed diabetics who have sustained a lot of irreversible damage, it slows down the progression of cardiovascular complications.[41]

Even nutrients commonly considered of marginal importance can have profound effects. One example is inositol, that much-neglected cofactor of the B complex. The normal concentration of inositol in the nerves of the human body is fifty times what it is in the blood.[42] Nature does not design such extreme gradients to no purpose. The high level of nerve inositol is essential for maintaining the conduction of nerve impulses. Without continuous conduction activity the nerve dies. One of the horrendous complications of diabetes is the gradual demise of nerves throughout the body. Especially feared is the death of the peripheral nerves, leading to pain and numbness of the hands and feet, arms and legs, progressing to the death of blood vessels and tissue, gangrene and amputation.

This process begins many years previously as a gradual but progressive deficiency of inositol in the nerves. We know it develops this way from animal experiments. In animals made diabetic artificially, nerve inositol declines rapidly. This causes a rapid decline in nerve conduction, threatening widespread death of the nerves. A simple dietary supplement of inositol *restores nerve function.*[43]

In human prediabetic and diabetic patients nerve conduction progressively declines. As the disease worsens, their toxic levels of blood sugar gradually poison the nerve bed. By an unknown mechanism, nerve inositol is displaced and excreted from the body in large quantities.[44] This continues to occur even in diabetics "controlled" by insulin, indicating beyond doubt that the disease is continuing to progress.

The important point for prevention is that the trend can be reversed. In 1977, at the University of Alabama Medical School, Dr. Rex Clements and his colleagues studied six women and fourteen men, all of whom had been diabetic at least nine years and were showing the usual peripheral nerve disorders. All had pain and numbness in the lower extremities. All showed profound disturbances in both sensory and motor nerve conduction. Half the patients were given a high-inositol diet and half a low-inositol diet for sixteen weeks. Then the diets were swapped, so that the low-inositol group got high inositol and vice versa for another sixteen weeks. The results were startling. For every patient, nerve conduction declined further when they were on the low-inositol diet. On the high-inositol diet, nerve conduction quickly and substantially improved and patients benefited accordingly.[45]

We know that the nerve damage in adult-onset diabetics begins years before any sign of diabetes appears, and that initially it is completely reversible.[46] So it makes very good sense for anyone with the slightest disturbance of sugar metabolism to use this nontoxic nutrient as insurance. The body of a healthy 150-pound man or woman produces up to 5 grams of inositol a day. In ill health you may make less than two grams. Yet a 150-pound body requires at least 9 grams of inositol daily. Even in good health, at least four grams a day must come from your food. If you eat the common American diet of white bread, milk, eggs and beef, with mainly frozen or canned vegetables and fruit, you will not get even one gram of inositol.

Some researchers object that dietary inositol increases blood inositol only a little in healthy people, no matter how much inositol they eat, so it cannot have much influence. The same argument applies to many dietary vitamins and minerals. It stems from erroneous concepts that still pervade medical science. Because blood gives good measures of a few bodily changes, some people believe it is a good measure of everything. It is not. For many substances the *bloodstream is simply a means of transport,* a highway carrying them to the muscles, organs or glands where they are stored and used. The fiftyfold concentration of inositol in the nerves compared with its concentration in the blood is just one of a *million* such gradients in the body.

We now know that many nutrients don't have to change blood levels much in order to have profound influences. Measuring their levels in the blood is like counting cars on the highway in the middle of the countryside in order to decide the number of cars there are in New York. The only accurate way to ascertain the number of cars in New York is to go to New York and count them. We cannot do this yet inside the human body. Meanwhile, dietary inositol is great insurance. The best natural source of dietary inositol is lecithin. It contains at least 1 gram of inositol per 100 grams (3½ oz). Then come wheat germ, rice germ, whole wheat, oatmeal and soya flour. Keep your intake ample.

Minerals Combat Diabetes

The essential minerals work only in interaction with vitamins and with each other. Medical science is only just realizing how *all* these nutrients together are involved directly or indirectly in maintaining normal sugar metabolism. Manganese, for example, is often deficient in people with poor glucose tolerance.[47] Without ample manganese the body cannot use the enzymes (biological catalysts which accelerate essential chemical reactions) necessary for the activity of choline, biotin, thiamin and Vitamin C. The result is multiple disorders, including the low production of acetylcholine leading to the impairment of nerve conduction that inevitably accompanies diabetes.

Chromium is *the* telling example. It was not until 1974 that Dr. Walter Mertz of the U.S. Department of Agriculture was able to persuade his colleagues (and the scientific world in general) that chromium permits insulin to act properly in the human body.[48] Now, we know that chromium is essential for insulin to maintain the delicate balance between hypoglycemia and hyperglycemia. Without it there is no way the body can handle sugar.

Because of the high level of processed carbohydrate in the American diet, body chromium is lost in the urine. Generally, it is not replaced, and the body gradually becomes depleted. Eggs, a usual American food, are often cited as being high in chromium. So they are, but unfortunately it is in a form that is not available to the human body. Raw fruits and vegetables contain some bioavailable chromium, but not enough. Unless your diet contains whole grains every day, it is likely to be deficient in chromium. Even then, the amount of chromium depends on the level in the soil on which the grains were grown. Each harvest uses up a lot of soil chromium along with other minerals. Much of the soil is now badly depleted. The fertilizers used to restore fertility contain only the minerals essential to good plant growth; that is, nitrogen, phosphorus and potassium. They do not contain the chromium, selenium or zinc essential for human health. Supplemental minerals are the only sure answer.

Chromium deficiency readily produces diabetes in animals, which can then be cured with chromium supplements.[49] Even in long-term diabetic patients, chromium supplements for a period of two to six months can improve glucose tolerance substantially.[50] The best sort of evidence that chromium is widely deficient in America, and thus may be a potent variable underlying our rising glucose intolerance and diabetes, is what happens when you give chromium supplements to apparently healthy Americans. In a typical study in 1981, Drs. Rebecca Riales and Margaret Albrink of the West Virginia University School of Medicine gave 200 mcg of chromium daily to twelve healthy men aged thirty-one to sixty for a period of six weeks.[51] At the start of the study their blood-insulin and blood-sugar levels were in the range considered normal for Americans. At the end of the study both levels dropped nearer to the range found in populations where diabetes is a rarity. Also, their high-density lipoprotein levels (HDLs) went up, indicating an additional beneficial effect on blood fats. It is likely that the levels we consider normal in America for blood insulin and blood sugar are actually a reflection of widespread borderline disorders of sugar metabolism, with dietary chromium deficiency as one of the major causes. With an appropriate supplement this condition is simple and inexpensive to correct. Diabetes, on the other hand, is incurable.

Exercise Combats Diabetes

A good diet and a complete vitamin and mineral supplement are two thirds of the diabetes prevention equation. The other third is regular exercise. Such exercise benefits prediabetics and even confirmed, insulin-dependent diabetics in several ways. First, exercise uses up excess blood sugar. It does this better in nondiabetics, because their insulin mechanism works to convert the sugar to energy. Prediabetics, however, tend to burn more fat when they exercise, because the body can't use its sugar properly. Nevertheless, this is of great benefit because, as we have seen, fat is one factor interfering with sugar metabolism. When prediabetics and diabetics exercise consistently, body fat and blood fats go down and the insulin mechanism recovers.[52] Even if no body fat is lost, twenty to thirty minutes of aerobic exercise a day causes blood fats and cholesterol to decline and glucose tolerance to improve.[53] Other studies have shown a beneficial reduction in blood insulin even with only three months of light exercise.[54]

In one recent study six nonobese diabetics with normal exercise electrocardiograms exercised three times a day for twenty to thirty minutes on an exercise bicycle at about half their maximum capacity. In all six, high blood-sugar levels dropped considerably, an average of 40 percent. In four of the patients, blood-glucose levels reliably dropped to normal on exercise days.[55] The beneficial effect of the exercise was not only during the exercise period but for at least twelve hours afterward. This finding parallels the evidence previously discussed in Chapter 8, that metabolic effects of exercise persist for up to fifteen hours afterward.

The diets of these patients were, of course, carefully controlled throughout, with frequent meals spaced to suit the exercise. Unlike many studies of aerobic exercise in insulin-dependent diabetics, no hypoglycemic episodes occurred during or after the exercise. If you are prediabetic or diabetic and wish to exercise both for improved general health and control of blood sugar, blood insulin and blood fats, then show this section and the accompanying references to your physician. On no account launch into an exercise program on your own. If you are not diabetic, but are in normal health and concerned to prevent the development of disturbances of sugar metabolism which could lead to diabetes, then this section provides additional support to what has been said in previous chapters, that the regular exercise part of the equation is essential to extended, healthy life.

CHAPTER 12

STOP POISONING YOURSELF

YOU CAN'T AVOID THE poisons in your air. But there are other poisons that cause degeneration and disease in all sorts of unlikely places, places where people commonly believe they are protected. There are protective laws aplenty; it's their implementation that is lacking. Not for want of trying, either. Sadly, no amount of conscientious work on the part of officials can protect us from runaway technology. It is up to you to protect yourself. Let's examine the miscellany of hazards against which self-protection is simple and effective.

Don't Drink the Water

Chemical poisoning of groundwater, the source of most drinking water, is the most dangerous pollution problem in America. Each year, about thirty outbreaks of diseases in the United States are traced to bacterial or chemical contamination of water supplies.[1] The Environmental Protection Agency (EPA) has collected evidence on fifty-five thousand chemical dumpholes across the nation which can leak their contents into the groundwater. Ironically, water purification for drinking by removal of natural hazards was first introduced in America in New Jersey in 1908. Today, in scientifically "enlightened" 1982, the water supply of Atlantic City, New Jersey, is being contaminated by chemicals leaking out of the infamous Price's Pit, a twenty-two-acre site of chemical dumping just six miles from the city.

The problem isn't a residue of the ignorance of yesteryear's industrialism. Price's Pit did not start to be a hazard until 1971. Then, in one and a half short years, nine million gallons of chemicals, including PCBs, deadly hydrocarbons and arsenic, were dumped there until authorities stepped in to stop it in 1972. Of course, they couldn't get out what had already been dumped. These poisons seeped away insidiously through the ground until suddenly they began appearing in one of the Atlantic City municipal wells nearly a mile away. Now, in 1982, seven of the twelve municipal wells have had to be closed down, leaving insufficient water to supply the city.

The same process is happening all over America. The tragedy is that groundwater pollution is technically irreversible. It may take as much as one hundred years for the ground to clean itself. And the carbon-filter methods used in an attempt to purify it are only marginally successful. Like most of the commercial filter systems offered for home use, they remove only large particles (above five microns in diameter, i.e., 1/5000 of an inch). Many industrial chemicals, viruses, pesticides, leached minerals and heavy metal particles are far smaller.

In the interests of human health, until 1981 the EPA was gaining a grip on the disposal of toxic wastes. Now, under new leadership and in the interests of economic recovery in America, many controls are being relaxed again. Each month industry produces two hundred million pounds of toxic wastes. While politicians argue, much of it is now being dumped without restraint.[2]

As a big-city dweller, you may have read that your water supply is free of such contamination. Unfortunately, chemical dumps are only a fraction of the story. The EPA has recently established a firm link between chlorinated tap water and cancer.[3] The very chemical, chlorine, which protects us by killing most waterborne infections, is now known to mix with chemical and organic wastes in the water to make a series of carcinogenic compounds called trihalomethanes. They are associated with cancer of the kidney, urinary tract, bladder, lymph nodes and brain. If you want to avoid trihalomethanes, the best advice is, don't drink the water. If it is cloudy, don't even wash in it. It may not make you sick today or tomorrow, but as we have seen, if it gradually induces cancer, your chance of survival is remote.

Because of these problems, the bottled water business is booming. Be warned. Labels saying "spring pure" or "natural spring fresh" are usually just filtered tap water. They are no better than your own. "Tested spring water" sounds better, but tested for what? There are over three hundred possible chemical contaminants. To test for them all regularly would push the price of water to thirty dollars a gallon. Words like "pure," "fresh," "natural" have no defined meaning. You can apply them freely to any product.

The Federal Trade Commission has fought a courageous but losing battle for years against misrepresentation in labeling. When you buy *any* food product, caveat emptor (let the buyer beware) applies more today than ever before in history. You can get manuals on testing your water from the EPA, Water Division, Washington, D.C. 20460. If you find your water wanting, forget home filters. The only really safe alternative is distilled water. You can buy it, of course, but it becomes a heavy item in more ways than one in the weekly shopping basket. My advice is to buy your own evaporation distiller. Then you can drink water freely, as you need to for good health. Expensive, but it will pay for itself in no time. The savings in health may be beyond price.

You Are Full of Food Additives

A grim joke in our lab is that the concentration of toxic chemicals in American mothers' milk has now reached such a level that it would be illegal to transport it across a state line in any other container. Statistics show that Americans eat nine pounds of chemical food additives a year. All are substances that do not occur naturally in foods. They are foreign, and therefore harmful, to the human body. Many are added to foods for trivial cosmetic reasons, to make cheese a little yellower, steak a little redder, fruit pies a little fruitier. If anyone tells you they are safe, don't believe it. Look for the vested interest, the commercial support of his or her laboratory, or the political puppeteer behind the scenes. The evidence against food additives is conclusive.[4]

Protective legislation is very difficult to pass, because food additives are tested singly. Alone, many show no harmful effects. Also, they are not tested long enough. Mutagenic (inducing genetic mutation) effects may not show until the next generation or the next. In combination, however, there is no longer any doubt that food additives lay silent foundations for the cancer or the heart disease you may suffer twenty years hence, or the deformity visited on your future children.

Only recently has the government accepted this "action at a distance" of toxic chemicals, with the irrefutable evidence of Agent Orange and the prospects of over $100 billion in lawsuits against it continuing long into the twenty-first century, as the children of children of Vietnam veterans continue to be born handicapped. Diethylstilbestrol (DES) is another prime example. In the 1960's this synthetic estrogen was prescribed for pregnant women to help prevent miscarriages. Silently, it worked its destruction on the growing female fetus, but the microscopic abnormalities caused to womb, cervix and vagina escaped the usual examinations. After puberty, however, *some fourteen to eighteen years later,* up to 90 percent of these girls developed cancer of the vagina or reproductive systems.[5]

For a decade the Food and Drug Administration (FDA) fought the food lobby to ban the use of DES as a growth stimulant in livestock, where it accumulates especially in the liver. Thankfully, since 1979 DES has been illegal. But are cases of cervical cancer going to turn up in the 1990's in the teenage daughters of women who ate lots of "nutritious" liver during pregnancy?

The FDA attempts to provide protection against additives under the Food, Drug and Cosmetic Act and the GRAS (generally recognized as safe) list of additives. Since 1959 many additives have been banned. But the evidence keeps coming in. The FDA's 1980 review of the latest studies on 415 additives on the GRAS list found twenty-four of doubtful safety, including monosodium glutamate, caffeine and butylated hydroxytoluene (BHT), chemicals that are added to a huge variety of foods. With caffeine suspect, you will have noticed the huge drive against it in advertising, in anticipation of a caffeine restriction, as coffee and soft-drink manufacturers scramble to reeducate the public palate so as to keep their shares of the beverage market. Incidentally, if you do switch to decaffeinated coffee, products that use water to remove the caffeine are the only safe buy.

In addition to additives, your body contains many residues of our out-of-control technology. Polychlorinated biphenyls (PCBs) are a prime example. These infamous industrial chemicals are used in everything from pesticides to electrical wiring. About four thousand tons a year escape into our water supply. They have got into all our meat, fish and milk. Today every nursing mother feeds them to her child at the breast.[6] Animal milks contain even more PCBs. High exposure causes permanent damage to the nervous system, especially in young children. Sweden put a *total* ban on PCBs in 1972. Because of their wide industrial utility, business avarice prevents America from taking the same sensible action.

The best way to avoid both deliberate and inadvertent contamination of your diet is to avoid all processed foods. Read labels assiduously. If chemicals abound in the contents list, don't buy the product. It is criminal to feed such "food" to children. Leave your nine pounds of additives on the supermarket shelf. If you, the public, vote with your pocketbooks against chemical additives, manufacturers will quickly make safer foods.

For contaminants you can't avoid, Vitamins C, E and the mineral selenium will help to protect you against substances that produce free radicals.[7] There is also growing evidence that B vitamins reduce the toxicity of pesticide residues.[8] The best protection, however, is a strong immune system nourished by complete vitamin and mineral supplementation.

Get the Lead Out of Your Life

Poisoning by toxic metal contamination of food leads not only to the fearsome diseases discussed in Chapter 3, but also to a host of other degenerative disorders. Recurrent gout and isolated joint arthritis, for example, have plagued men of the southeastern United States for a century.[9] It is a case of "So your sins shall seek ye out." These disorders are saturnine gout, caused by drinking hootch whiskey, which is usually heavily contaminated with lead. The lead damages the kidneys and prevents uric-acid excretion, which then deposits as crystals in the joints of the lower extremities. Continued imbibing over many years brings death by kidney failure.

Unfortunately, you don't have to sin to suffer lead poisoning. Because of lead pollution, the bodies of most Americans today carry over fifty times more lead than in the past, causing fatigue, memory loss, impaired judgment and depression.[10] We get heavily leaded from the seams of food cans. Recently, Dr. D. G. Mitchell and his colleagues bought 122 canned foods and beverages over-the-counter in upstate New York.[11] The average lead content was 80 mcg per pound of food, with some canned baby foods showing over 100 mcg lead. The FDA now considers that there may be no *safe* level of lead. Some baby foods now come in welded cans, but in general, feeding canned food or drink to an infant is dangerous. The lead damages developing bones, brain and organs. Recent studies show that many cases of mental retardation and learning disabilities are linked with high levels of lead in the children with these conditions.[12] The switch to aluminum cans is no improvement. Aluminum is almost as poisonous as lead and harder for the body to get rid of. Aluminum's effects are more insidious than lead's. They take twenty years to show.[13]

Refrigeration May Not Prevent Spoilage

The shining ranks of open refrigerators in our supermarkets give us a misplaced confidence that our food is being protected. Often it is not. All low-acid foods, such as meat, fish, cheese and milk products, are highly susceptible to bacteriological spoilage. They have to be stored at below 28° F for safety. Thermometers *attached* to supermarket refrigerators may show below this figure. These are misleading, because the exposed surfaces of the food may be as much as 10° warmer. If food is held for days in an open refrigerator where a thermometer placed *on top* of the food shows higher than 28° F, then bacteria, yeasts and molds are growing freely. Don't buy it.

The same applies to the expiration dates stamped on cartons. These dates apply only to properly refrigerated food. Dating implies care and is therefore a good selling point in an increasingly health-conscious market. So, numerous products are now dated that are held on the open shelves above refrigerated cabinets, which appear to be part of the cold store but do little to maintain foods at low temperature. If meat, fish or cheese products can be held this way without spoilage, then they contain too much preservative to be good for you.

Overcoming spoilage problems by irradiating food with Cobalt 60 is the popular new solution. The half-life of the irradiation is supposedly so brief and the dose so minute that when you get to eat the food, there is no radioactivity left. We are examining this novel procedure, and frankly, do not believe it. With our emphasis that science cannot beat nature but can only cooperate with her, I thought we might be getting a little paranoid. So I asked six leading medical scientists here at Rockefeller University the simple question, "Would you eat food that had been irradiated with Cobalt 60 to preserve it?" Five said "No" and one said "Only if there was nothing else."

Even the Vegetables . . .

We have noted already that vegetables of the nightshade family contain solanine, a poisonous chemical called a glycoalkaloid with many detrimental effects on the body. For example, Dr. Norman Childers of Rutgers University has shown conclusively that eating potatoes, tomatoes, red and green peppers, eggplant and paprika, or any foods containing them, is associated with arthritic pain.[14] What is often neglected in discussions of Dr. Childers' work is the huge variation in solanine content. *Solanum tuberosum,* the common potato, is a major offender. Potatoes grown close to the surface, where they can develop chlorophyll, may have ten times the solanine of deep-grown varieties. So the folk warning against green potatoes is correct.

Unfortunately, new vegetable varieties are developed for rapid growth, uniform size, ease of picking and other commercial considerations. The promotion of human health is last on the list. Some of the newer potatoes, such as the Houma, Oromonte, Cascade and Chieftain varieties, have almost twice the solanine of traditional varieties such as Red Pontiac or Irish Cobbler. If you have arthritic pain, gout, bursitis or just general achiness, and you can't give up your potatoes, avoid the high-solanine types. Some new varieties, such as Norgold Russet, Penobscot and Shurchip, are low in solanine.[15] Incidentally, if you grow your own vegetables, low-solanine varieties are available in all the nightshade plants. The American Medical Association maintains a list.

The innocent-looking parsnip is also toxic. Parsnips contain three poisonous chemicals called psoralens. Even at moderate levels psoralens are acutely toxic and can cause mutation and cancer.[16] You can't get rid of psoralens by peeling and cooking. One serving of parsnips (3 oz) can give you 5 mg of psoralens, a toxic amount. The common practice of feeding parsnips to infants in canned baby food is a tragedy. In 1980 a medical review of psoralens in parsnips concluded that any unnecessary exposure to them should be avoided.[17]

Plants of the genus *Brassica* include most varieties of cabbage, turnips, kale, rutabaga, watercress and rapeseed. They contain chemicals called thioglucosides, which damage thyroid function and can cause goiter. The toxic effects of thioglucosides on livestock are so bad that rapeseed meal used for fodder has to be specially treated to reduce thioglucoside activity.[18] If you have a known or suspected thyroid insufficiency, avoid eating these foods raw. Cooking destroys the toxins.

Plants high in oxalic acid should also be avoided, especially as you get to middle age and beyond. Spinach, rhubarb and cocoa beans (including all chocolate), and to a lesser extent broccoli, asparagus, coffee and tea, interfere badly with calcium absorption by forming insoluble salts with the calcium in food, rendering it unavailable to the body. Incidentally, high-fat diets do this also by combining with calcium to form a sort of rancid soap in the intestine which cannot be absorbed. One major cause of the widespread epidemic of osteoporosis (fragile bones that have lost calcium) in certain areas of America may be the popularity of calcium inhibiting foods like spinach in the diet. And giving children chocolate milk to ensure they get their calcium is ludicrous.

A final point concerns vegetable oils. Most cooking oils are heated during processing, which destroys their natural antioxidants. Advertisements that say they contain no cholesterol or saturated fats obscure the problem that they have lost their protection against oxidation. Fed to animals, processed vegetable oils produce diseases from muscular dystrophy[19] to sudden death from heart attack.[20] Manufacturers can sell processed vegetable oils for human use because we are supposed to be protected by the wide variety of our diets. Far better to protect yourself by using cold-pressed oils. Be sure the label says "cold-pressed," rather than using meaningless terms like "pure," "natural," "unrefined," "unprocessed" or "uncooked." If you eat out a lot, Vitamins C, E and the mineral selenium will protect you.

Medicines Are Toxic

America is the worst country in the world for pill-popping. Daily we are bombarded by advertisements for ineffective nostrums for everything from headache to hemorrhoids. Fewer than one thousand chemicals are used in the three hundred thousand over-the-counter remedies sold in America. Studies by the Food and Drug Administration show that there is *no evidence of efficacy* in two thirds of the uses for which these chemicals are sold. For one third of ingredients, there is no evidence even that they are safe.[21]

The Federal Trade Commission can't protect you, though it does its best. It made Warner Lambert spend ten million dollars to correct the false advertising that Listerine could relieve colds. Of course, you paid for it. And the FTC has Anacin on the run for implying it can relieve tension. But usually by the time the FTC can act, the ad is finished and the damage done.

Prescription drugs are worse, because they are more powerful. In 1973 the then-director of the FDA's Bureau of Drugs, Dr. Henry Simmons, testified to the government that overprescription is a major American health hazard, and that each year 1.5 million people are admitted to a hospital because of drug reactions. He stated also that one patient in five has his or her hospital stay *doubled* as a result of drug reactions.[22] In 1979 the Surgeon General repeated the warnings about overprescription.[23] Reading these reports and others,[24] and seeing the results in hospitals and clinics, I have been forced to the sad conclusion that, too often, prescription is a procedure used to fill in the time while waiting for natural healing processes to occur, and has only detrimental effects.

Good work in rooting out the drug rot in our society is now being done by many organizations, such as the Center for Science in the Public Interest in Washington, D.C., Public Citizen, Inc., the consumer arm of the Nader organization, and consumer advocates such as John Stossel, the New York consumer editor of WCBS-TV. The bottom line is not to take any form of drug, even aspirin, unless absolutely unavoidable. If presently you swallow them by the handful, you are not to blame. Pharmaceutical conglomerates spend billions of dollars indoctrinating us that every sniffle or twinge spells health disaster without their nostrums. Prescription drugs are sometimes necessary for the really sick. But for any of the myriad minor ills, to which the malnourished body is easy prey, over-the-counter nostrums simply add a further toxic burden to an already weakened system. Historians of medicine will look back in disbelief at a technology capable of putting men on the moon whose approach to everyday health was still rooted in alchemy.

Perhaps unwittingly, television health programs are also to blame. In October 1981 the *New England Journal of Medicine* published a special preview of the U.S. Public Health Service report, *Health and Medicine on Television.* The report concluded that portrayals of dramatic successes in dire diseases gave a misleading optimistic view of the effectiveness of medical treatment. The report concluded that such portrayals promote a misplaced confidence in doctors to provide cures, and breed lack of concern about prevention, the basis of effective health care.[25] The only sure protection against disease is a strong, well-nourished body. Get your body into that state, and you will wonder how you ever tolerated the way you were before.

EPILOGUE

I CANNOT WRITE A summary chapter. This whole book is but a brief summary with a few brief examples. Discoveries in medical science over the last decade show that former beliefs about diet, nutrition, exercise and aging are incorrect. We know now that the application of nutrition science to prevent degenerative disease will soon be saving many millions of people from countless years of suffering.

We know now that the seeds of degenerative disease are planted early in life, even while the person feels perfectly well. And all the medical tests for disease will show nothing amiss. Without adequate nutrition there is no way to prevent these degenerative processes from becoming established in the young body. And without vitamin and mineral supplements there is no way today to get adequate nutrition.

Unfortunately, like any progress that overturns old beliefs, and threatens the commercial structure that those beliefs support, the new knowledge of nutrition is meeting harsh criticism from vested interests and the tame professionals who take their funds and sing their tunes. Against these powerful forces of commerce, books such as this one are essential to direct the public away from reliance on medical treatment of disease *after* it has ravaged the body, and toward individual responsibility for health maintenance to prevent disease from gaining a foothold.

Some may judge it premature to release this information to the public. Not yet enough experiments, not enough data, not the technology available, they may say. They are mistaken. Their thinking has become obscured by the complex mechanics of science. Concepts which advance human understanding do not depend on technology. It is the other way around. Concepts create the studies and the technical means for their application. Forming a new concept is a creative act as much as is the writing of a symphony. Does that not make science an art? Indeed, it does, and like all art, its finest works do not depend on experiments, data bases or technological breakthroughs. They stem from an individual's leap of comprehension in which is perceived a new pattern underlying that mass of changing sensations which we crudely call reality.

It is true that some of the crucial nutrition experiments are still going on. It is true that others are not yet begun. But it will be twenty-five years before these studies are complete. Meanwhile, we know that nutritional supplements are essential to healthy functioning in today's environment. We know that each person has different vitamin and mineral needs. And we know that those needs can be calculated so as to provide a complete supplement tailored to the individual. And if you would live beyond the common span, we know that daily exercise is an essential component of the health formula.

But there are benefits far beyond health if you follow the advice in this book, benefits we have had neither time nor space to discuss. The healthy body produces increased quantities of substances called endorphins, biochemicals which are responsible for our feelings of well-being. It is not too far a stretch of the evidence to infer that optimum health is therefore a major basis of human happiness.

Happiness and well-being promote the flow of all those singular virtues which set humans apart from their animal kin. Happiness and well-being promote that pursuit of emotional bonds which hold us in love and cooperation with each other.

Happiness and well-being promote that pursuit of excellence which will take us to the stars.

But there is a further, greater benefit. While the world remains full of sickness, we will not overcome the bestial urges of our animal heritage, those emotional sicknesses which spawn the violence, war and outrage that shadow our lives. Only when man is truly a healthy animal will we be able to cast off those shackles of disordered emotion, will we be able to pursue those human virtues collectively called nobility. Only then will we be able to appreciate as a group the differences between justice and vindictiveness, between dignity and pomp, between morality and convention, between discipline and servility, between beauty and decoration, and between love and convenience. To bring optimum health to the mass of our peoples is to put in place the foundation of the noblest feat to which the human mind can aspire—to bring peace to this earth.

APPENDIX 1

HEALTH FACTS OR HOCUS-POCUS

WELL-KNOWN nutrition researcher Victor Herbert of the State University of New York rages that vitamin supplements are a waste of time.[1] Eminent scientist Roger Williams of the University of Texas claims they are vital.[2] Small wonder many people are bewildered by the diametrically opposed views of different sections of the scientific community. Who is right? Unless you understand what constitutes scientific evidence, it is impossible to evaluate health information. Yet without this evaluation you cannot prevent disease. Let's see what makes a scientific fact.

Evaluating the Evidence

There are five main types of study which provide the evidence to support the concepts of science: anecdote, case study, case series, unblinded trial and double-blind controlled trial. The weakest is anecdote. For example, a man is found to have high cholesterol. He tells his doctor he is going to eat spinach every day for a month to lower it, because he's read that Popeye doesn't have heart trouble, or for some other offbeat reason. At the end of the month his cholesterol is down 15 percent, a significant drop in terms of cardiovascular risk. Our jubilant hero believes Popeye forever. But cholesterol can vary by at least 15 percent without treatment, depending on weight, sleep, stress, exercise, alcohol, infection and a host of other factors. It is very unlikely that this man's cholesterol drop was caused by the spinach.

Such anecdotes and testimonials fill the pages of nutrition books, health-food magazines and newspaper advertisements. *All* of them should be ignored. They are just handbills for snake-oil hucksters. The value of anecdotal observations is only to provide science with hunches to be scientifically tested by controlled experiments before anything can be said. Over 99 percent of such hunches prove to be dead wrong.

All the nutrition books and media reports that refer to this study or that, at this or that university, by this or that professor, *but which fail to give a reference to a scientific report where the details can be examined,* are useless too. These reports often exaggerate, misinterpret or distort the findings. The data reported are often preliminary and unreliable. Sometimes the study has been junked because it didn't work after all. Other times the studies simply don't exist. If a publication does not give you the scientific references, ignore it.

The "controlled case study" is better. Such information can be found in medical and scientific journals, where all papers submitted are reviewed by other scientists before being accepted for publication. Authors are not paid for their work and the rejection rate is high for all the major journals. Thus, a lot of suspicious or shoddy studies are weeded out. Unlike the Popeye fables, good case studies involve measurements and controls which can be repeated by other scientists. It is this quality of being replicable which makes case studies useful. In themselves they do not provide evidence of any general truth. They are merely a better form of hunch. So, for the purpose of deciding your own health strategy, ignore them.

The "case series" studies are still better. These have standardized measurement procedures and repeated observations and controls applied to each of a series of cases. To carry on with the spinach hypothesis, each case gets measured repeatedly, *before* giving the spinach, *during* the period of eating spinach and again *after* the spinach is stopped. If cholesterol falls for every case only during the period of spinach-eating, then we have some *fair* evidence. Case series used to be the backbone of clinical medicine and applied human science until their faults were recognized. There is just too much room for unconscious (and deliberate) manipulation of the data.

Unfortunately, scientific committees often think they can overcome such bias by making a case series larger, as if size converts bad data into good. Like many of us, they are fooled by the common emphasis that big is better and monstrous is divine. A lovely example is given by eminent nutrition specialist Professor Ancel Keys. A massive case series of 750,000 survey questionnaires was used by the actuary of Metropolitan Life Insurance to show that premature death from heart disease is directly related to overweight. The sheer size and cost of the study made it look very impressive. Closer investigation, however, shows that the study was carried out by nonprofessional volunteers, and subjects were not weighed at all but were simply asked their weight and height.[3] The huge potential for error and manipulation makes the study useless as a source of health evidence. Good science demands more rigorous standards.

The "unblinded trial" ("unblinded" because everyone knows what's going on) is the minimum standard of evidence you should accept as a basis for protecting your own health. In such experiments the responses of an experimental group, the group that gets the spinach, are compared with those of a control group, which gets no spinach but otherwise is treated identically. If cholesterol drops for the experimental subjects but doesn't for the controls, then Popeye wins. Sometimes the experimental group acts as its own control, with the spinach being given for a period, then removed for a period, then given again. If the cholesterol of the whole group goes down, then up, then down again correspondingly, we have reasonable evidence of a spinach effect. (No, spinach doesn't work.)

The most acceptable evidence is the "double-blind controlled trial." In its simplest form there is an experimental group and a control group, and neither scientists nor patients know which group gets the spinach. One group gets real spinach (ground up and put into capsules) and the other group gets capsules of green-colored milk powder. Which is which is filed under code numbers in a computer. The key to the code is often put in a safe-deposit vault. No one can match the code to the cholesterol counts until after the whole study is over. So, ideally, no one can manipulate anything. This is the sort of evidence we want. If Popeye could pass this test, we should all eat spinach.

A final word on evidence concerns the use of animals in nutrition studies. Many are inappropriate. Rabbits, for example, have been used to test whether meat in the diet causes atherosclerosis. These are silly studies, because rabbits are natural vegetarians. Feeding them on meat disturbs their whole system. Yet cats fed on meat show no changes at all, as you would expect because cats are natural carnivores. Neither animal is a good model for man, who is a natural omnivore. Scientific reports often note these limitations, but by the time they reach the media, all restrictions are abandoned and you see reports of mouse experiments, for example, under headlines like "New B Vitamin Prevents Gray Hair." Pure hogwash!

Whom to Believe

If we lived in an ideal world, evidence from double-blind nutrition experiments on human subjects would provide a fine base for your health strategy. But, alas, vested interests can distort anything. Whenever you read new studies about nutrition, vitamins, minerals or health practices, ask yourself immediately, who is doing the reporting and who funded the work? Much of what you see and read about nutrition and health is subtly underwritten by pharmaceutical houses and food-processing conglomerates. Publicity about new findings may come from a "medical information bureau" or "medical news service" or some other cover name designed by a commercial enterprise to impress science reporters, editors, broadcasters and, through them, the public. Often the well-meaning health reporter is steered by the company to researchers doing studies for it, studies that are purely company funded and company controlled.[4]

Worse, there are also unscrupulous researchers who turn in just the sort of results the sponsoring companies want, without ever conducting proper studies at all. They get very large fees![5] After many complaints in the early 1970's from scientists who just could not believe the gee-whiz in drug company publicity releases, the Food and Drug Administration set up an investigation headed by Dr. Francis Kelsey, the courageous scientist who also blew the whistle on thalidomide. Of fifty physicians investigated, sixteen were found to have supplied false information. One of the investigating team commented wryly that when he saw data on drug effects on the testicles of *female* rats, he began to get suspicious! In another study, tissue slides from a reported series of animals were shown to be all from one animal—very economical.[6] The FDA investigation found many such errors and falsifications. Your only protection is to have access to the research report.

Even the top of the scientific tree is a bit wilted. In order to fund their research programs, most universities, including Harvard, Rockefeller, Stanford, UCLA and MIT must take corporate money. Understandable. What is difficult to accept is why distinguished scientists such as Dr. Frederick Stare, head of Harvard's nutrition department, consider themselves unbiased in testifying to congressional Food and Drug Administration hearings on behalf of the very corporations (such as the Kellogg Company and Carnation Milk) that make major grants to their departments.[7] When such testimony can affect the health of millions of Americans, it is essential that such corporate ties automatically disqualify the scientist just as they disqualify the juror or the government official. "Forgetting" a thousand-dollar gift was enough for President Reagan's National Security Adviser Allen to lose his job.

The government is aware of the problem. Examining public misinformation about nutrition, in 1969 the White House Conference on Food, Nutrition and Health concluded, "The American people falsely believe that they are well protected both by government and by the ethics of commerce."[8] The number of nutrition scientists who receive major financial support from the food and drug conglomerates is enormous. So be very cautious before accepting what they say in their syndicated columns, in television interviews or press conferences.

Even physicians are not above corporate bias. Consider, for example, the American Medical Association (AMA) debacle over disbanding its own council on drugs. Professor John Adriani, professor of surgery at Tulane, told the Senate Monopolies Subcommittee in 1973 that the council, which was composed of tough physicians determined not to be influenced by vested interests, was disbanded because its findings were displeasing the pharmaceutical industry, and the AMA did not want to lose pharmaceutical advertising revenue in its journals. Adriani said: "For a number of years the AMA, which derives a large part of its income for its annual budget from advertising of drugs, has been a captive of and beholden to the pharmaceutical industry."[9]

The AMA has since produced a number of drug manuals. And in the 1,470 pages of the latest *AMA Drug Evaluations*[10] are listed numerous drugs with instructions for use by physicians which the FDA has long declared ineffective and therefore illegal, but which it has failed to have banned because of legal maneuvers by the drug companies. A full list of these *non*health products can be obtained from Public Citizen Inc., the Consumer arm of the Ralph Nader organization.

Do not be afraid to pursue such cited sources of evidence. Scientists and physicians are often arrogant to the point of ridicule in pretending that the intelligent layman cannot evaluate medical evidence. If you have to struggle with the unfamiliar jargon, remember that the evaluation of one thoughtful individual is worth the unthinking authority of a posse of professors. It is your health and your responsibility, and if you think it takes too much time, trouble and expense to preserve it—try disease. And write and tell me if you find my analysis wanting. Even without bias, scientists are as fallible as anyone, and I would like to get my bloopers out of the next edition.

MICHAEL COLGAN
The Rockefeller University
1230 York Avenue
New York, N.Y. 10021

May 1982

APPENDIX 2

EATING TO PREVENT HERPES

The following are foods which can trigger Herpes 1 and 2 and some other viral infections of mucous membranes, foods that are neutral in relation to these ailments and foods which should be eaten during active infection:

Forbidden Foods (especially during active infection)
- Chocolate and all foods containing chocolate (e.g., candy and cocoa)
- Corn and popcorn and all products containing corn
- Brown rice
- White rice
- Canned peas and beans
- Peanuts and all peanut products
- Cashews
- Pecans
- Walnuts
- Most grains not listed as acceptable
- All processed foods containing preservatives
- Red wine
- Cheese foods and processed cheeses
- Tomatoes and all citrus fruits if canker sores are present

Eat in Moderation (especially during active infection)
- Red meat

Breakfast cereals
All bread
All flour
Crackers
Macaroni
Noodles and spaghetti
Pancakes
Pretzels
Cakes and sweets
Coconut
Almonds
Chick peas
Mung beans and sprouts
Lentils
Refined sugar
Rye
Barley
Wheat
Oats
Alfalfa sprouts

Can Be Eaten at All Times

Wheat germ
Cucumbers
Peas (not canned)
Eggplant
Yellow and green beans
Carrots
Honey
Cabbage
Beets
Spices
Bamboo shoots
Fruits and berries (except tomatoes and citrus as noted)
Artichokes
Margarine

- Mushrooms
- Butter
- Pickles
- Lettuce
- Radishes
- Vegetable oils
- Salad dressings
- Mayonnaise
- Coffee and tea
- Onions and garlic
- Squash and pumpkins
- White wine
- Soups without grains
- Soybeans and soybean products
- Worcestershire sauce
- Lima beans

Increase Intake During Active Infection

- All cheeses except processed
- Yogurt
- Kefir
- Cottage cheese
- Sour cream
- Milk
- Eggs
- All fish
- All shellfish
- All other seafood
- Chicken
- Turkey
- Potatoes

REFERENCES

SPACE RESTRICTIONS MAKE it possible to cite only a fraction of the references used in writing this book. For some points made, one or more references are cited which exemplify the evidence available.

References are arranged by chapter. Names of journals are abbreviated in the normal fashion for medical literature. To assist readers unfamiliar with these abbreviations, the full names and abbreviations of major journals cited are given below.

Acta Diabetica Latina	*Acta Diabetica Lat.*
Advances in Experimental Medicine and Biology	*Adv. in Ex. Med. and Biol.*
American Heart Journal	*Am. Heart J.*
American Journal of Clinical Nutrition	*Am. J. Clin. Nutr.*
American Journal of Clinical Pathology	*Am. J. Clin. Pathol.*
American Journal of Digestive Diseases	*Am. J. Dig. Dis.*
American Journal of Epidemiology	*Am. J. Epidemiology*
American Journal of Medicine	*Am. J. Med.*
American Journal of Pathology	*Am. J. Pathol.*
American Journal of Physiology	*Am. J. Physiol.*
American Journal of Psychiatry	*Am J. Psychiatry*
American Journal of Roentgenology	*AJR*
American Society for Experimental Biology	*Am. Soc. Exp. Biol.*
American Surgery	*Am. Surg.*

Annals of Internal Medicine	*Ann. Intern. Med.*
Annals of the New York Academy of Science	*Ann. N.Y. Acad. Sci.*
Annals of Surgery	*Ann. Surg.*
Annual Review of Medicine	*Ann. Rev. Med.*
Archives of Biochemistry	*Arch. Biochem.*
Archives of Environmental Health	*Arch. Environ. Health*
Archives of General Psychiatry	*Arch. Gen. Psychiatry*
Archives of Internal Medicine	*Arch. Intern. Med.*
Archives of Neurology	*Arch. Neurol.*
Archives of Surgery	*Arch. Surg.*
Biochemical and Biophysical Research Communications	*Biochem., Biophys. Res. Comm.*
Biological Psychiatry	*Biol. Psychiatry*
Biological Trace Element Research	*Biol. Trace Element Res.*
Brain Research	*Brain Res.*
British Heart Journal	*Br. Heart J.*
British Journal of Cancer	*Br. J. Cancer*
British Journal of Clinical Pharmacology	*Br. J. Clin. Pharmacol.*
British Journal of Industrial Medicine	*Br. J. Indust. Med.*
British Medical Journal	*Br. Med. J.*
Bulletin of the New York Academy of Medicine	*Bull. N.Y. Acad. Med.*
Canadian Medical Association Journal	*Can. Med. Assoc. J.*
Cancer Research	*Canc. Res.*
Circulation: Journal of the American Heart Association	*Circulation*
Circulation Research	*Circ. Res.*
Clinical and Experimental Immunology	*Clin. Exp. Immun.*
Clinical Medicine	*Clin. Med.*
Clinical Pharmacology and Therapeutics	*Clin. Pharmacol. Ther.*
Clinical Research	*Clin. Res.*
Clinical Science and Molecular Medicine	*Clin. Sci. Mol. Med.*
Environmental Health Perspectives	*Environ. Health Perspect.*
Experimental Cell Research	*Exp. Cell Res.*
Federal Proceedings	*Fed. Proc.*
International Journal of Epidemiology	*Int. J. Epidem.*
International Journal of Radiation Biology	*Int. J. Radiation Biol.*

International Journal of Vitamin and Nutrition Research	*Int. J. Vitam. Nutr. Res.*
Internationale Zeitschrift für Angewandte Physiologie Einschliesslich Arbeitphysiologic	*Int. Z. Angew. Physiol.*
Journal of Argriculture and Food Chemistry	*J. Agric. Food Chem.*
JAMA: Journal of the American Medical Association	*JAMA*
Journal of the American Dietetic Association	*J. Am. Diet. Assoc.*
Journal of the American Geriatrics Society	*J. Amer. Geriatr. Soc.*
Journal of Applied Nutrition	*J. Appl. Nutr.*
Journal of Applied Physiology	*J. Appl. Physiol.*
Journal of Atherosclerosis Research	*J. Atherosclerosis Res.*
Journal of Chronic Diseases	*J. Chron. Dis.*
Journal of Clinical Endocrinology and Metabolism	*J. Clin. Endocrinol. Metab.*
Journal of Clinical Investigation	*J. Clin. Invest.*
Journal of Clinical Pathology	*J. Clin. Pathol.*
Journal of Gerontology	*J. Gerontol.*
Journal of Infectious Diseases	*J. Infect. Dis.*
Journal of Inorganic Biochemistry	*Bioinorganic Chem.*
Journal of the National Cancer Institute	*J. Nat'l. Cancer Inst.*
Journal of Nutrition	*J. Nutr.*
Journal of Nutritional Science and Vitaminology	*J. Nutr. Sci. Vitaminol.*
Journal of Occupational Medicine	*J. Occup. Med.*
Journal of the Pharmaceutical Society of Japan	*Japanese J. Pharm.*
Journal of Psychosomatic Research	*J. Phsychosom. Res.*
Mayo Clinic Proceedings	*Mayo Clin. Proc.*
Mechanisms of Aging and Development	*Mech. Aging Dev.*
Medical Clinics of North America	*Med. Clin. North Am.*
Medical Journal of Australia	*Med. J. Aust.*
Medicine and Science in Sports	*Med. Sci. Sports*
Metabolism, Clinical and Experimental	*Metab. Clin. Exp.*
New England Journal of Medicine	*N. Eng. J. Med.*
New Zealand Medical Journal	*New Zeal. Med. J.*
Nutrition Reviews	*Nutr. Reviews*
Physiological Reviews	*Phys. Rev.*
Proceedings of the National Academy of Science, U.S.A.	*Proc. Nat. Acad. Sci., U.S.A.*

Proceedings of the Nutrition Society	*Proc. Nutr. Soc.*
Proceedings of the Society for Experimental Biology and Medicine	*Proc. Soc. Exp. Biol. Med.*
Research Quarterly, American Alliance for Health, Physical Education, and Recreation	*Res. Q. Amer. Assoc. Health Phys.*
Scandinavian Journal of Gastroenterology	*Scand. J. Gastroenterology*
Schweizerische Medizinische Wochenschrift	*Schweiz. Med. Wschr.*
Science of the Total Environment	*Sci. Total Environment*
Scottish Medical Journal	*Scott. Med. J.*
South African Medical Journal	*South African Med. J.*
Surgery, Gynecology and Obstetrics	*Surg. Gyn. Obstet.*

Chapter 1

1. R. I. Levy, Address to the National Institutes of Health, November 27, 1979, mimeographed.

2. National Cancer Institute, *National Cancer Institute Monograph 57,* NIH Publication No. 81-2330 (Bethesda, Md.: June 1981).

3. The Surgeon General, *Healthy People: The Surgeon General's Report on Health Promotion and Disease Prevention,* DHEW, Pub. Nos. 79-55071 and 79-55071A (Washington, D.C.: 1979).

4. U.S. National Center for Health Statistics, *Mortality for Leading Causes of Death in the United States 1977,* DHEW (Hyattsville, Md.: 1981).

5. The Surgeon General, *op. cit.*

6. R. Dubos, and J. Dubos, *The White Plague: Tuberculosis, Man and Society* (Boston: Little Brown, 1953), passim.

7. G. F. McCleary, *Infant Mortality and Infant Milk Depots* (London: King, 1905).

8. R. R. Porter, Paper presented to the British Association for the Advancement of Science (London: BAAS, 1971).

9. The Surgeon General, *op. cit.* p. 6.

10. Ibid. p. viii.

11. C. E. Butterworth, *JAMA,* Vol. 230, (1974), p. 879.

12. H. G. Mather, *Br. Med. J.,* Vol. 3 (1971), p. 334.

13. N. Wade, *Science,* Vol. 180 (1973), p. 1038. *See also* N. Wade, *Science,* Vol. 179, (1973), p. 775.

14. U.S. National Center for Health Statistics, *Vital Statistics of the United States,* DHEW Volumes for 1973–1980. (Rockville, Md.: 1975).

15. U.S. National Center for Health Statistics, *Facts of Life and Death.* DHEW (Hyattsville, Md.: 1979).

16. N. Worthington, "National Health Expenditures 1929–74," *Social Security Bulletin,* (Feb. 1975).

17. *The Budget of the United States, Fiscal Year 1981* (Washington, D.C.: USGPO 1981).

18. U.S. National Center for Health Statistics, Rockville, Md., personal communication, October 1981.

19. U.S. House of Representatives Committee on Ways and Means, *Basic Facts on the Health Industry* (Washington, D.C.: USGPO, 1971), passim.

20. J. Ferry-Pierret and S. Karsenty, *Practiques Médicales et Système Hospitalier,* (Paris: Cerebe, 1974), passim. *See also* E. Friedson, ed., *The Hospital in Modern Society* (New York: Free Press, 1963).

21. D. Kotelchuck, ed., *Prognosis Negative: Crisis in the Health Care System* (New York: Random House, 1976), passim. *See also* I. Illich, *Medical Nemesis* (New York: Bantam Books, 1976), passim.

22. U.S. Dept. of Health, Education and Welfare, *Report of the Secretary's Commission on Medical Malpractice* (Washington, D.C.: 1973), passim.

23. J. T. McLamb, and R. R. Huntley, *Southern Med. J.,* Vol. 60 (1967), p. 469.

24. New South Wales Health Commission, "Survey of Hospital Treatment," mimeographed (Sydney: 1978).

25. U.S. National Center for Health Statistics, *Limitation of Activity and Mobility Due to Chronic Conditions, United States 1972,* DHEW, Series 10 (Rockville, Md.: 1974).

26. The Surgeon General, *op. cit.*

27. U.S. National Center For Health Statistics, *Vital Statistics of the United States,* Volumes for 1970–1980 (Rockville, Md.: 1975).

28. A. Keys, *Circulation,* Vol. 41 (1970), Supp. 1.

29. The Surgeon General, *op. cit.*

30. Ibid.

31. Ibid. pp. 56–67.

32. American Cancer Society, "Cancer Statistics, 1982," *Ca—A Cancer Journal for Clinicians,* Vol. 32 (1982), p. 26.

33. C. L. Meinert et al., *Diabetes,* Vol. 19 (1970), Supp. 2, p. 789. *See also* G. Knatterud et al., *JAMA,* Vol. 217 (1971), p. 777.

34. The Surgeon General, *op. cit.* p. 68.

35. Ibid.

36. Association for Children with Learning Disabilities, *Taking the First Step to Solving Learning Problems* (Pittsburgh: mimeographed), 1980.

37. Ongoing study at the University of California reported in J. D. Beasley, *The Impact of Nutrition on the Health of Americans,* A report to the Ford Foundation by The Medicine and Nutrition Project (Annandale-on-Hudson, N.Y.: Bard College, 1981).

38. National Swedish Board of Health and Welfare, *Psykisk Halsovard 1* (Stockholm: Liber forlag, 1978).

Chapter 2

1. V. Herbert, *Nutrition Cultism* (Philadelphia: George F. Stickley, 1980), p. 147.

2. *First Health and Nutrition Examination Survey, United States 1971–72,* DHEW, Publication 76-1219-1 (Rockville, Md.: 1976).

3. *Ten State Nutritional Survey, United States,* DHEW, Pub. Nos. 72-8130-1, 2, 3 (Rockville, Md.: 1972), passim.

4. T. K. Murray, *Proc. Western Hemisphere Nutrition Congress IV,* eds. N. Selvey and P. L. White, American Medical Association (Acton, Mass.: Publishing Sciences, 1975), p. 331.

5. C. M. Leevy et al., *Am. J. Clin. Nutr.,* Vol. 17 (1965), p. 259.

6. A. J. Bollet and S. Owens, *Am. J. Clin. Nutr.,* Vol. 26 (1973), p. 931.

7. B. R. Bistrian et al., *JAMA,* Vol. 230 (1974), p. 858.

8. C. E. Butterworth, *Nutrition Today,* Vol. 9 (1974), p. 4.

9. C. E. Butterworth, *JAMA,* Vol. 230 (1974), p. 879.

10. Ibid.

11. L. M. Klevay et al., *JAMA,* Vol. 241 (1979), p. 1916.

12. B. R. Bistrian et al., *JAMA,* Vol. 235 (1976), p. 1567.

13. M. E. Shils, *Nutrition in the 1980's: Constraints on Our Knowledge,* eds. N. Selvey and P. L. White, American Medical Association (New York: Allen R. Liss, 1981), p. 71.

14. R. L. Weinsier et al., *Am. J. Clin. Nutr.,* Vol. 32 (1979), p. 418.

15. B. Peterkin, *Nutrition in the 1980's: Constraints on Our Knowledge,* p. 59.

16. American Medical Association Council on Foods and Nutrition, ed., *Nutrients in Processed Foods* (Acton, Mass.: Publishing Sciences Group, 1974), passim. *See also* B. K. Watt and A. L. Merill, *Composition of Foods* (Washington, D.C.: U.S. Dept. of Agriculture, 1963), passim.

17. B. Patrias and O. Olson, *J. Agric. and Food Chem.,* Vol. 15 (1967), p. 448.

18. E. J. Underwood, *Trace Elements in Human and Animal Nutrition,* 4th ed. (New York: Academic Press, 1977), passim.

19. F. R. Senti, *Nutrients in Processed Foods,* ed. American Medical Association Council on Foods and Nutrition (Acton, Mass.: Publishing Sciences Group, 1974), p. 39.

20. R. E. Hein and I. J. Hutchings, *Nutrients in Processed Foods,* ed. American Medical Association Council on Foods and Nutrition (Acton, Mass.: Publishing Sciences Group, 1974).

21. H. A. Schroeder, *Am. J. Clin. Nutr.,* Vol. 24 (1971), p. 562.

22. Senti, *op. cit.*

23. L. Brewster and M. Jacobson, *The Changing American Diet* (Washington, D.C.: Center for Science in the Public Interest, 1978).

24. J. Mayer, *Science,* Vol. 188 (1975), p. 566.

25. W. Mertz, *Science,* Vol. 213 (1981), p. 1332.

26. S. Soskin and R. Levine, *Modern Nutrition in Health and Disease,* 3rd ed., eds. M. G. Wohl and R. S. Goodheart (Philadelphia: Lea & Febiger, 1964), p. 208.

27. R. J. Williams, *Orthomolecular Psychiatry,* eds. D. Hawkins and L. Pauling (San Francisco: W. H. Freeman, 1973), p. 316.

28. R. J. Williams and R. B. Pelton, *Proc. Nat. Acad. Sci., U.S.A.,* Vol. 55 (1966), p. 126.

29. National Research Council, Food and Nutrition Board, *Toward Healthful Diets* (Washington, D.C.: Academy of Sciences 1980).

30. Watt & Merrill, *op. cit.*

31. Ibid.

32. E. D. Fries, *Circulation,* Vol. 53 (1976), p. 589.

33. J. D. Beasley, *The Impact of Nutrition on the Health of Americans,* A report to the Ford Foundation by The Medicine and Nutrition Project (Annandale-on-Hudson, N.Y.: Bard College, 1981).

34. M. Biskind, *Am. J. Digest. Dis.,* Vol. 20 (1953), p. 57.

35. The Surgeon General, *Healthy People: The Surgeon General's Report on Health Promotion and Disease Prevention,* DHEW, Pub. Nos. 79-55071 and 79-55071A (Washington, D.C.: 1979), passim.

36. Biskind, *op. cit.*

37. L. D. Ostrander, *Circulation,* Vol. 30 (1964), p. 67.

38. M. Colgan, "Effects of Vitamin and Mineral Supplementation on Physiology and Performance of Athletes and in Adjunctive Treatment of Certain Mental Disorders and Human Degenerative Diseases," (Paper given at Rockefeller University, March 1981).

Chapter 3

1. J. Warren, *Journal of the Royal Society of Medicine,* Vol. 74 (January 1981), p. 42.

2. A fair summary is given in "Those Costly Annual Physicals," *Consumer Reports* (October 1980), p. 601.

3. L. Kuller et al., *Circulation,* Vol. 34 (1966), p. 1056.

4. "Those Costly Annual Physicals," *Consumer Reports* (October 1980), p. 601.

5. G. S. Siegel, *Arch Environ. Health,* Vol. 13 (1966), p. 292. *See also* P. D. Clote, *Antologia,* (Cuernavaca: Cidoc, 1974), p. A8.

6. W. O. Spitzer, *Can. Med. Assoc. J.,* Vol. 121 (1979), p. 1193.

7. The Surgeon General, *Healthy People: The Surgeon General's Report on Health Promotion and Disease Prevention,* DHEW, Pub. Nos. 79-55071 and 79-55071A (Washington, D.C.: 1979), p. 14.

8. R. L. Weinsier et al., *Am. J. Clin. Nutr.,* Vol. 32 (1979), p. 418.

9. M. E. Shils, *Nutrition in the 1980's: Constraints on Our Knowledge* (New York: Alan R. Liss, 1981).

10. W. H. Sebrell, *Vitam. Horm.,* Vol. 22 (1964), p. 875.

11. F. Stare, quoted in *Hunger U.S.A.* (Washington, D.C.: The New Community Press, 1968), p. 40.

12. *The 1969 White House Conference on Food, Nutrition and Health, Final Report* (Washington, D.C.: USGPO, 1970), p. 159.

13. Editorial, "Nutrition Education in Medical Faculties," *Am. J. Clin. Nutr.,* Vol. 24 (1971), p. 1399.

14. J. Schorr, quoted in M. Brelove, *The Wall Street Journal,* January 12, 1971.

15. M. Latham, quoted in *Time,* December 16, 1972.

16. *Priorities for the Use of Resources in Medicine,* DHEW Report No. (NIH) 77-1288 (Washington, D.C.: USGPO, 1976), passim. *See also* R. J. Carlson, *The End of Medicine* (New York: Wiley, 1975), passim; M. Lalonde, *A New Perspective on the Health of Canadians* (Ottawa: Govt. of Canada, 1974), passim.

17. A. E. Shaefer, *Am. J. Clin. Nutr.,* Vol. 34 (1981), p. 961.

18. W. Mertz, *Science,* Vol. 213 (1981), p. 1332. *See also* E. J. Underwood, *Trace Elements in Human and Animal Nutrition,* 4th ed. (New York: Academic Press, 1977); National Research Council Food and Nutrition Board, *Recommended Dietary Allowances,* 9th ed. (Washington, D.C.: National Academy of Sciences, 1980); and O. A. Levander and L. Cheng, eds., *Micronutrient Interactions: Vitamins, Minerals and Hazardous Elements,* Ann. N.Y. Acad. Sciences, Vol. 355 (New York: New York Academy of Sciences, 1980).

19. Underwood, *op. cit.*

20. K. Schwarz et al., *Biochem., Biophys. Res. Comm.,* Vol. 40 (1970), p. 22.

21. Underwood, *op. cit.*

22. F. H. Nielson et al., *Am. Soc. Exp. Biol.,* Vol. 34 (1975), p. 923.

23. M. Philips and A. Baetz, eds., *Diet and Resistance to Disease, Advances in Experimental Medicine and Biology,* Vol. 35. (New York: Plenum Press, 1981).

24. R. E. Hodges et al., in Levander & Cheng, eds., *op. cit.* p. 58.

25. J. M. Navia and S. S. Harris, in Levander & Cheng, eds., *op. cit.* p. 45.

26. J. C. Smith, in Levander & Cheng, eds., *op. cit.* p. 62.

27. C. J. McClain et al., *Alcoholism: Clin. Exper. Res.,* Vol. 3 (1979), p. 135.

28. J. S. McLester and W. J. Darby, *Nutrition and Diet in Health and Disease* (Philadelphia: W. B. Saunders, 1952).

29. H. E. Sauberlich, in Levander & Cheng, eds., *op. cit.* p. 80.

30. S. R. Lynch and J. O. Cook, in Levander & Cheng, eds., *op. cit.* p. 32.

31. J. K. Davis, in Levander & Cheng, eds., *op. cit.* p. 130.

32. F. H. Nielson, in Levander & Cheng, eds., *op. cit.* p. 152.

33. J. C. B. Grant, *An Atlas of Anatomy,* 6th ed. (Baltimore: Williams & Wilkins, 1972).

34. R. J. Williams, *Biochemical Individuality* (New York: Wiley, 1956), passim.

35. R. J. Williams et al., *Lancet,* Vol. 1 (1950), p. 287.

36. R. J. Williams and G. Deason, *Proc. Nat. Acad. Sci., U.S.A.,* Vol. 57 (1967), p. 1638.

37. S. Lewin, *Vitamin C: Its Molecular Biology and Medical Potential* (London: Academic Press, 1976), passim.

38. A. E. Harper, *N.Y. State J. Med.,* Vol. 79 (1979), p. 806.

39. Lewin, *op. cit.*

40. E. Cameron, L. Pauling and B. E. Leibovitz, *Cancer Res.,* Vol. 39 (1979), p. 663. *See also* B. E. Leibovitz, B. V. Siegel, *Diet and Resistance to Disease,* eds. M. Philips and A. Baetz (New York: Plenum Press, 1981).

41. R. J. Williams, *Protein and Amino Acid Nutrition,* ed. A. A. Albanese (New York: Academic Press, 1959), p. 45.

42. Ibid. *See also* R. J. Williams, *Physicians' Handbook of Nutritional Science* (Springfield, Ill.: Thomas, 1975).

43. R. J. Williams, *Physicians' Handbook.*

44. W. F. Bodmer, *Nature* (London), Vol. 237 (1972), p. 139. *See also* Philips and Baetz, *op. cit.*

45. Philips and Baetz, *op. cit.*

46. J. Dausset, *Science,* Vol. 213 (1981), p. 1474.

47. B. O. Barnes and L. Galton, *Hypothyroidism: The Unsuspected Illness* (New York: Crowell, 1976).

48. R. B. Gillie, *Human Physiology and the Environment in Health and Disease,* ed. A. J. Vander (San Francisco: W. H. Freeman, 1976), p. 21.

49. L. D. Greenberg and J. F. Rinehard, *Fed. Proc.,* Vol. 7 (1948), p. 157. *See also* L. D. Greenberg et al., *Arch. Biochem.,* Vol. 21 (1949), p. 237.

50. J. F. Meller and J. M. Iancono, *Am. J. Clin. Nutr.,* Vol. 12 (1963), p. 358.

51. S. R. Tannebaum and W. Mergens, in Levander & Cheng, eds., *op. cit.* p. 267.

52. L. M. Klevay et al., *JAMA,* Vol. 241 (1979), p. 1916. *See also* J. M. Holden et al., *J. Am. Diet. Assoc.,* Vol. 75 (1979), p. 23.

53. D. Oberleas, *Proc. West. Hemisphere Nutrition Congress IV,* eds. N. Selvey and P. L. White, American Medical Association (Acton, Mass.: Publishing Sciences Group, 1975), p. 156.

54. C. C. Pfeiffer, *Mental and Elemental Nutrients: A Physician's Guide to Health Care* (New Canaan, Conn.: Keats, 1975).

55. V. F. Fairbanks et al., eds., *Clinical Disorders of Iron Metabolism,* 2nd ed. (New York: Grune & Stratton, 1971).

56. P. Sturgeon and A. Shoden, *Am. J. Clin. Nutr.,* Vol. 24 (1975), p. 469.

57. E. R. Monsen et al., *Am. J. Clin. Nutr.,* Vol. 20 (1967), p. 842.

58. V. F. Fairbanks, *op. cit.*

59. S. J. Baker and E. M. De Maeyer, *Am. J. Clin. Nutr.,* Vol. 32 (1979), p. 368.

60. The Surgeon General, *The 1979 Surgeon General's Report on Smoking and Health,* DHEW, Pub. No. 017-000-0218-0 (Washington, D.C.: 1979), passim.

61. The Surgeon General, *The Health Consequences of Smoking: The Changing Cigarette,* Dept. of Health and Human Services (Washington, D.C.: 1981).

62. J. L. Repace, *Bull. N.Y. Acad. Med.* (in press, 1982).

63. O. Pelletier, *Am. J. Clin. Nutr.,* Vol. 23 (1970), p. 520.

64. *First Health and Nutrition Examination Survey, United States 1971–72,* DHEW, Pub. No. 76-1219-1: (Rockville, Md.:1976).

65. Pelletier, *op. cit.*

66. An accurate summary of effects of alcohol is given in *The Harvard Medical School Health Letter,* Vol. 7 (1981), p. 2.

67. Editorial, "Screening for alcoholism," *Lancet,* Vol. 2 (1980), p. 1117.

68. D. F. Horrobin, *Med. Hypotheses,* Vol. 6 (1980), p. 929. *See also* D. F. Horrobin and M. S. Manku, *Br. Med. J.,* Vol. 1 (1980), p. 1363.

69. Food and Drug Administration, *Drug Bulletin* (July 1980).

70. The Surgeon General, *Healthy People,* p. 101.

71. M. R. Spivey et al., in Levander & Cheng, eds., *op. cit.* p. 249. *See also* H. H. Sandstead, in Levander & Cheng, eds., *op. cit.* p. 282.

72. H. H. Sandstead, *op. cit.*

73. G. F. Nordberg, ed., *Effects and Dose Response Relationships of Toxic Metals* (Amsterdam: Elsevier, 1976).

74. Spivey, in Levander & Cheng, *op. cit.*

75. K. E. Mason and J. O. Young, *Selenium in Biomedicine,* eds. O. H. Muth et al. (Westport, Conn.: Avi, 1967).

76. D. R. Crapper et al., *Brain,* Vol. 99 (1976), p. 67.
77. H. Spencer et al., in Levander & Cheng, eds., *op. cit.* p. 181.
78. L. Fishbein, *Sci. Total Environ.,* Vol. 2 (1974), p. 341.
79. J. H. Koeman et al., *Sci. Total Environ.,* Vol. 3 (1975), p. 279.
80. H. E. Ganther, in Levander & Cheng, eds., *op. cit.* p. 212.
81. L. Kosta et al., *Nature* (London), Vol. 254 (1975), p. 238.
82. *Report: Comm. Biol. Effects Atmos. Pollutants* (Washington, D.C.: National Academy of Sciences, 1971), passim.
83. Food and Drug Administration, Washington, D.C., personal communication, February 12, 1982.
84. *Consumer Reports* (July 1981), p. 376.
85. H. G. Petering, in Levander & Cheng, eds., *op. cit.* p. 298.
86. K. R. Mahaffey and J. I. Rader, in Levander & Cheng, eds., *op. cit.* p. 285.
87. Ibid.
88. O. A. Levander et al., in Levander & Cheng, eds., *op. cit.* p. 227.

Chapter 4

1. L. Levi, *Int. J. Mental Health,* Vol. 9 (1981), p. 9.
2. C. E. Finch and L. Hayflick, *Handbook of the Biology of Aging* (New York: Van Nostrand, 1977).
3. M. Gould, *Science 81* (April 1981), p. 29.
4. K. N. Jeejeebhoy et al., *Clin. Res.,* Vol. 23 (1975), p. 636.
5. R. Holliday et al., *Science,* Vol. 198 (1977), p. 366.
6. R. L. Walford, *Am. J. Clin. Pathol.,* Vol. 74 (1980), p. 247.
7. P. D. Wood, *Med. Sci. Sports* (in press, 1981). *See also* K. H. Sidney et al., *Am. J. Clin. Nutr.,* Vol. 30 (1977), p. 326.
8. Wood, *op. cit. See also* E. L. Smith, et al., *AJR,* Vol. 126 (1976), p. 1297; and T. Kavanagh and R. J. Shephard, *The Marathon: Physiological, Medical, Epidemiological and Psychological Studies,* ed. P. Milvy (New York: New York Academy of Sciences, 1977), p. 656.
9. P. D. Wood and W. L. Haskell, *Lipids,* Vol. 14 (1979), p. 417. *See also* A. S. Leon and H. Blackburn, in Milvy, ed., *op. cit.* p. 561.
10. A. S. Leon & H. Blackburn, in Milvy, ed., *op. cit. See also* Kavanagh & Shephard, in Milvy, ed., *op. cit.*
11. L. B. Oskai, *Nutrition in the 1980's: Constraints on Our Knowledge,* eds. N. Selvey and P. L. White (New York: Alan R. Liss, 1981), p. 383
12. Kavanagh & Shephard in Milvy, ed., *op. cit.*
13. T. J. Carlow et al., *Neurology,* Vol. 28 (1978), p. 390. *See also* J. Griest, *J. Psychosom. Res.,* Vol. 22 (1978), p. 259

14. A. P. Polednak, *The Longevity of Athletes* (Springfield Ill.: C. C. Thomas, 1979).
15. L. Moorehouse, *The Physiology of Exercise,* 7th ed. (St. Louis: Mosby, 1976).
16. C. Rose and M. Cohen, in Milvy, ed., *op. cit.* p. 671.
17. Kavanagh & Shephard, in Milvy, ed., *op. cit.*
18. P. M. Fenton and E. J. Brassey, *The Case for Exercise,* Sports Council Research Working Paper No. 8 (London: Sports Council, 1979).
19. S. P. Modak et al., *Exp. Cell Res.,* Vol. 65 (1971), p. 289.
20. R. W. Hart and R. B. Setlow, *Proc. Nat. Acad. Sci., U.S.A.,* Vol. 71 (1974), p. 2165.
21. J. Smith-Sonneborn, *Science,* Vol. 203 (1979), p. 1115.
22. G. S. Smith and R. Walford, *Nature,* Vol. 270 (1977), p. 727.
23. R. L. Walford and K. Bergmann, *Tissue Antigens,* Vol. 14 (1979), p. 336.
24. U. Paffenholz, *Mech. Aging Dev.,* Vol. 7 (1978), p. 131.
25. R. L. Walford, *The Immunologic Theory of Aging* (Copenhagen: Minksgaard, 1969).
26. J. D. Mathews et al., *Lancet,* Vol. 1 (1973), p. 754.
27. N. Cohen ed., *The Reticuloendothelial System,* Vol. 5 (New York: Plenum Press, 1980).
28. Walford, *op. cit.*
29. R. G. Cutler *J. Human Evolution,* Vol. 5 (1976), p. 169.
30. A. Michelson et al., *Superoxide and Superoxide Dismutases* (New York: Academic Press, 1977).
31. B. E. Leibovitz and B. V. Siegel, *J. Gerontol.,* Vol. 35 (1980), p. 45. *See also* A. L. Tappel, *Micronutrient Interactions: Vitamins, Minerals and Hazardous Elements,* eds. O. A. Levander and L. Cheng, *Ann. N.Y. Acad. Sciences,* Vol. 355 (New York: New York Academy of Sciences, 1980), p. 18.
32. R. Badiello and M. Jielden, *Int. J. Radiation Biol.,* Vol. 17 (1970), p. 1.
33. A. L. Tappel et al., *J. Gerontol.,* Vol. 28 (1973), p. 415.
34. L. Packer and J. R. Smith, *Advances in Experimental Medicine and Biology,* Vol. 61, eds. V. J. Cristofalo et al. (New York: Plenum Press, 1975).
35. L. Packer and J. R. Smith, *Proc. Nat. Acad. Sci., U.S.A.,* Vol. 74 (1977), p. 1640.
36. E. V. Barnett et al., *Immunological Aspects of Aging,* eds. D. Segre and L. Smith (New York: Dekker, 1980).
37. R. L. Walford, *Am. J. Clin. Pathol.,* Vol. 74 (1980), p. 247.
38. J. S. Milne et al., *Br. Med. J.,* Vol. 4 (1971), p. 383. *See also* A. V. Pisciotta et al., *Nature,* Vol. 215 (1967), p. 193; and M. Brook and J. J. Grimshaw, *Am. J. Clin Nutr.,* Vol. 21 (1968), p. 1254.
39. G. M. G. Barton and O. S. Roath, *Int. J. Vitam. Nutr. Res.,* Vol. 46

(1976), p. 271; C. W. M. Wilson and H. S. Loh, *Lancet,* Vol. 1 (1973), p. 1058; and M. Green and S. W. M. Wilson, *Br. J. Clin. Pharmacol.,* Vol. 2 (1975), p. 369.

40. R. Hume and E. Weyers, *Scott. Med. J.,* Vol. 18 (1973), p. 3.

41. C. W. M. Wilson and H. S. Loh, *op. cit.*

42. O. Pelletier, *Am. J. Clin. Nutr.,* Vol. 23 (1970), p. 520.

43. B. V. Siegel and J. I. Morton, *Experientia,* Vol. 33 (1977), p. 393.

44. R. Anderson et al., *Am. J. Clin. Nutr.* Vol. 33 (1980), p. 71. *See also* R. H. Yonemoto, *Int. J. Vitam, Nutr. Res.,* Vol. (1979), Supp. 19.

45. S. Lewin, *Vitamin C: Its Molecular Biology and Medical Potential* (London: Academic, 1976).

46. Ibid. *See also* W. R. Thomas and P. G. Holt, *Clin. Exp. Immun.,* Vol. 32 (1978), p. 370; L. Pauling, *Medical Tribune,* (March 24, 1976), p. 1; and I. M. Baird et al., *Am. J. Clin. Nutr.,* Vol. 32 (1979), p. 1686.

47. B. V. Siegel and J. I. Morton, *op. cit. See also* R. Anderson, *op. cit.*

48. A. E. Axelrod and J. Pruzansky, *Ann. N.Y. Acad. Sci.,* Vol. 63 (1955), p. 202. *See also* A. E. Axelrod and S. Hopper, *J. Nutr.,* Vol. 72 (1960), p. 325.

49. V. Herbert and K. C. Das, *Vitamins and Hormones,* Vol. 34, eds. P. L. Minson et al. (New York: Academic Press, 1976), p. 1.

50. S. W. Thenen, *J. Nutr.,* Vol. 108 (1978), p. 836.

51. K. C. Haltalin et al., *J. Infect. Dis.,* Vol. 121 (1970), p. 275.

52. A. Lavoie et al., *Clin. Sci. Mol. Med.,* Vol. 47 (1974), p. 617.

53. R. P. Tengerdy, *Diet and Resistance to Disease, Advances in Ex. Med. and Biol.,* Vol. 135, eds. M. Philips and A. Baetz (New York: Plenum Press, 1981), p. 27.

54. R. H. Heinzerling et al., *Infection and Immunity,* Vol. 10 (1974), p. 1292.

55. R. P. Tengerdy, in Philips & Baetz, eds., *op. cit.* p. 40.

56. H. H. Sandstead, *Am. J. Clin. Nutr.,* Vol. 26 (1973), p. 1251.

57. P. J. Fraker and R. W. Leucke, in M. Philips & A. Baetz, eds., *op. cit.* p. 107.

58. C. M. McCay, *J. Nutr.,* Vol. 18 (1939), p. 1.

59. M. H. Ross, *Nutrition and Aging,* ed. M. Winick (New York: Wiley, 1976).

60. B. N. Berg, *J. Nutr.,* Vol. 71 (1960), p. 242.

61. M. H. Ross, *Am. J. Clin. Nutr.,* Vol. 25 (1972), p. 834.

62. C. H. Barrows and G. Kokkonen, *Growth,* Vol. 39 (1975), p. 525.

63. R. H. Weindruch et al., *Fed. Proc.,* Vol. 38 (1979), p. 2007.

64. S. Freud, *Collected Works of Sigmund Freud,* ed. and trans. J. Strachey (London: Hogarth Press, 1955), passim.

65. J. H. Pincus and G. J. Tucker, *Behavioral Neurology* (London: Oxford University Press, 1974). *See also* D. Hawkins and L. Pauling, eds., *Orthomolecular Psychiatry* (San Francisco: W. H. Freeman, 1973).

66. National Institute on Aging, *JAMA,* Vol. 244 (1980), p. 259.
67. R. Hall et al., *Arch. Gen. Psychiatry* (September 1980), p. 471.
68. N. Wade, *Science,* Vol. 179 (1973), p. 775.
69. The Surgeon General, *Healthy People: The Surgeon General's Report on Health Promotion and Disease Prevention,* DHEW, Pub. Nos. 79-55071 and 79-55071A, (Washington, D.C.: 1979), p. 75.
70. Ibid. p. 155.
71. S. Garb, *Undesirable Drug Interactions 1974–1975* (New York: Springer, 1975), passim.
72. D. A. Drachman and J. Leavitt, *Arch. Neurol.,* Vol. 30 (1974), p. 113. *See also* D. A. Drachman, *Neurology,* Vol. 27 (1977), p. 783.
73. M. J. Hirsch and R. J. Wurtman, *Science,* Vol. 202 (1978), p. 222.
74. W. D. Boyd et al., *Lancet,* Vol. 2 (1977), p. 711.
75. S. H. Ferris, *Science,* Vol. 205 (1979), p. 1039.
76. R. C. Mohs et al., *Am. J. Psychiatry,* Vol. 136 (1979), p. 1275.
77. J. L. Signoret et al., *Lancet,* Vol. 2 (1978), p. 837.
78. R. W. Bartrop, et al., *Lancet,* Vol. 1 (1977), p. 834.
79. J. Bjorksten, *Longevity—A Quest* (Madison, Wisc: Bjorksten Research Foundation, 1981), p. 230.

Chapter 5

1. L. Moorehouse, *The Physiology of Exercise,* 7th ed. (St. Louis: Mosby, 1976).
2. W. Van Huss, Paper given at the National American College of Sports Medicine Conference, May 1974, Knoxville, Tennessee.
3. D. Talbot, *Sport and Fitness Instruction* (June 1974).
4. Some of the substances listed have shown minor effects in animals. But even supposing the same effects in humans, the amounts used in the animal studies would require you to eat them by the jarful every day to get an equivalent effect. Most products sold as "Vitamin B_{15}" contain nothing but lysine, glycine and calcium gluconate. Some contain disopropylammonium dichloroacetate (a minor stimulant). A few contain n-n-dimethylglycine (a tertiary amino acid involved in choline metabolism in the body). There is new evidence that this latter substance enhances immune function. We are awaiting the results of further studies now under way. *See* C. D. Graber et al., *J. Infect. Dis.,* Vol. 143 (1981), p. 101.
5. C. Klafs and D. Arnheim, *Modern Principles of Athletic Training,* 4th ed. (St. Louis: Mosby, 1977).
6. R. Early and B. Carlson, *Int. Z. Angew. Physiol.,* Vol. 27 (1969), p. 43.
7. J. O. Steel, *Med. J. Aust.,* Vol. 2 (1970), p. 728.

8. E. Hilsendager and R. Karpovich, *Res. Q. Amer. Assoc. Health Phys. Ed.,* Vol. 35 (1964), p. 389. *See also* H. Montoye et al., *J. Appl. Physiol,* Vol. 7 (1955), p. 589.

9. C. Shaffer, *Am. J. Clin. Nutr.,* Vol. 23 (1970), p. 27.

10. K. Boddy et al., *Clin. Sci. Mol. Med.,* Vol. 46 (1974), p. 449.

11. K. J. Stone and B. H. Townsley, *Biochem. J.,* Vol. 131 (1973), p. 611.

12. H. Howald et al., *Ann. N.Y. Acad. Sci.,* Vol. 258 (1975), p. 458.

13. T. Van Itallie, *Nutrition Today,* Vol. 3 (1968), p. 3.

14. E. Buskirk and E. Haymes, *Women and Sport: A National Research Conference,* ed. D. Harris (Penn State University, 1972).

15. Howald et al., *op. cit. See also* G. O. Grey et al., *JAMA,* Vol. 211 (1970), p. 105; P. Rasch et al., *Sport zarzliche Praxis,* Vol. 5 (1962), p. 10; and D. A. Bailey et al., *Am. J. Clin. Nutr.,* Vol. 23 (1970), p. 905.

16. J. Marks, *The Vitamins in Health and Disease* (London: Churchill, 1968).

17. T. W. Bunch, *Mayo Clin. Proc.,* Vol. 55 (1980), p. 113.

18. C. Zauner and W. Updyke, *Swimming Technique,* Vol. 10 (1973), p. 61.

19. N. Yakovlev and V. Rogozkin, Paper presented at the National Conference of American College Sports Medicine, New Orleans, May 1975.

20. M. Colgan, *Biol. Psychiatry* (submitted, 1982).

21. M. Gliedman and C. Roth, *Unexpected Minority: Handicapped Children in America* (Carnegie Council Report, New York: Harcourt Brace, 1980).

22. Association of Children with Learning Disabilities, *Taking the First Step to Solving Learning Problems* (mimeograph, Pittsburgh, 1980).

23. B. Rimland, *Orthomolecular Psychiatry,* eds. D. Hawkins and L. Pauling (New York: W. H. Freeman, 1973), p. 513.

24. B. Rimland et al., *Am. J. Psychiatry,* Vol. 135 (1978), p. 472.

25. M. Coleman et al., *Biol. Psychiatry,* Vol. 14 (1979), p. 708.

26. B. Rimland, Publication No. 39, Institute for Child Behavior Research, 1980, 4157 Adams Avenue, San Diego, California 92116. The vitamin/mineral formula for use with autistic children is Super Nu-Thera, produced by Kirkman Laboratories, Box 3929, Portland, Oregon 97208.

27. B. Rimland and G. E. Larson, Institute for Child Behavior Research, 4157 Adams Avenue, San Diego, California 92116.

28. National Institute of Health Consensus Development Conference, *Defined Diets and Hyperactivity* (January 1982), pp. 13–15.

29. R. F. Harrell et al., *Proc. Nat. Acad. Sci., U.S.A.,* Vol. 78 (1981), p. 574.

30. American Academy of Pediatricians, "AAP Policy Statement," *AAP News and Comment* (August 1981), p. 4.

31. R. F. Harrell, *Metabolism,* Vol. 5 (1956), p. 555.

32. M. B. Stoch and P. M. Smythe, *Archives of Disease in Childhood,* Vol. 38 (1963), p. 546.

33. National Academy of Sciences, *Ability Tests: Uses, Consequences and Controversies* (Washington, D.C.: National Academy Press, 1982).

34. J. L. McGaugh, *Animal Memory,* eds. W. K. Honig and P.H.R. James (New York: Academic Press, 1972).

35. K. L. Davis et al., *Science,* Vol. 201 (1978), p. 272.

36. N. Sitaram et al., *Science,* Vol. 201 (1978), p. 274.

37. L. Solyom et al., *J. Gerontol.,* Vol. 22 (1967), p. 1.

38. Sitaram, *op. cit.*

Chapter 7

1. G. D. Novelli, *Phys. Rev.,* Vol. 33 (1953), p. 525.

2. P. C. Fry, *J. Nutr. Sci, Vitaminol.,* Vol. 22 (1976), p. 339.

3. National Research Council Food and Nutrition Board, *Recommended Dietary Allowances,* 9th ed. (Washington, D.C.: National Academy of Sciences, 1980).

4. Ibid.

5. E. P. Ralli and M. E. Dumm, *Vit. Horm. N.Y.,* Vol. 11 (1953), p. 133.

6. Nat. Res. Council Food and Nutrition Board, *op. cit.*

7. B. K. Watt and A. Merrill, *Composition of Foods* (Washington, D.C.: USDA, 1963).

8. AMA Dept. of Drugs, *AMA Drug Evaluations,* 4th ed. (Littleton, Mass.: American Medical Association, 1980).

9. Ibid.

10. Ibid.

11. C. C. Pfeiffer, *Mental and Elemental Nutrients: A Physician's Guide to Health Care* (New Canaan, Conn.: Keats, 1975).

12. AMA Dept. of Drugs, *op. cit.*

13. Pfeiffer, *op. cit.*

14. Ibid.

15. AMA Dept. of Drugs, *op. cit.*

16. J. P. Onjour, *Int. J. Vitam. Nutr. Res.,* Vol. 47 (1977), p. 107.

17. K. L. Davis et al., *Science,* Vol. 201 (1978), p. 272.

18. F. R. Klenner, *J. Appl. Nutr.,* Vol. 23 (1971), p. 61.

19. AMA Dept. of Drugs, *op. cit.*

20. "Report of the Committee on International Dietary Allowances," *Nutrition Abstracts and Reviews,* Vol. 45 (1975), pp. 2 and 89.

21. AMA Dept of Drugs, *op. cit.*

22. Ibid.

23. C. C. Pfeiffer, *Zinc and Other Micronutrients* (New Canaan, Conn.: Keats, 1978).

24. R. Riales and M. J. Albrink, *Am. J. Clin. Nutr.,* Vol. 34 (1981), p. 2670.

25. Nat. Res. Council Food and Nutrition Board, *Recommended Dietary Allowances,* 7th ed. (Washington, D.C.: National Academy of Sciences, 1968), p. 61.

26. Ibid., 9th ed.

27. Ibid., 7th ed.

28. E. I. Hamilton and M. J. Minski, *Sci. Total Environ.,* Vol. 4 (1972), p. 375.

29. AMA Dept. of Drugs, *op. cit.*

30. Ibid.

31. F. W. Sunderman, *Am. J. Clin. Path.,* Vol. 35 (1961), p. 203.

32. E. I. Hamilton and M. J. Minski, *op. cit.*

33. C. Kagen, *Lancet,* Vol. 1 (1974), p. 137. *See also* R. S. Griffith, *Dermatologica,* Vol. 156 (1978), p. 257.

34. H. Fisher et al., *J. Atherosclerosis Res.,* Vol. 7 (1967), p. 381.

35. D. Y. Graham, *N. Eng. J. Med.,* Vol. 296 (1977), p. 1314.

36. Ibid.

37. K. D. Lee and R. Huemer, *Japanese J. Pharm.,* Vol. 21 (1970), p. 299. *See also* K. Takagi et al., *Japanese J. Pharm.,* Vol. 22 (1972), p. 339; and H. Theonen et al., *Japanese J. Pharm.,* Vol. 27 (1977), p. 445.

38. A. Aslan et al., *Research on Novocaine Therapy in Old Age* (New York: Medical Consultants Bureau, 1959).

39. S. Cohen and K. S. Ditman, *Psychosomatics,* Vol. 14 (1974), p. 15. *See also* W.W.K. Zung et al., *Psychosomatics,* Vol. 15 (1974), p. 127.

40. Aslan, *op. cit.*

41. P. R. Dallman, *Nutrition in the 1980's: Constraints on Our Knowledge,* eds. N. Selvey and P. L. White (New York: Alan R. Liss, 1981), p. 87.

Chapter 8

1. S. Abraham and C. L. Johnson, *Vital and Health Statistics of the National Center for Health Statistics,* DHEW, Pub. No. 51 (Hyattsville, Md.: 1979).

2. Association of Life Insurance Medical Directors of America and the Actuarial Society of America, personal communications, February 1982. *See also* E. A. Lew and L. Garfinkel, *J. Chron. Dis.,* Vol. 32 (1979), p. 563.

3. A. Keys, *Nutrition in the 1980's: Constraints on Our Knowledge,* eds. N. Selvey and P. L. White (New York: Alan R. Liss, 1981).

4. R. Edelman, in Selvey & White, eds., *op. cit. See also* E. H. Ahrens and W. E. Connor, *Am. J. Clin. Nutr.,* Vol. 32 (1979), p. 2621; and E. L. Bierman, *Nutrition and Aging,* ed. M. Winick (New York: Wiley, 1976).

5. A. Angel, *Can. Med. Assoc. J.,* Vol. 119 (1978), p. 1401.

6. The Surgeon General, *Healthy People: The Surgeon General's Report on Health Promotion and Disease Prevention,* DHEW, Pub. Nos. 79-55071 and 79-5501A (Washington, D.C.: 1979).

7. R. K. Chandra, *Fed. Proc.,* Vol. 39 (1980), p. 3088.

8. K. J. Printen et al., *Am. Surg.,* Vol. 41 (1975), p. 483. *See also* National Academy of Sciences, *Ann. Surg.,* Vol. 160 (1964), p. 32; and P. J. Cruse and R. Foord, *Arch. Surg.,* Vol. 107 (1973), p. 206.

9. V. V. Tracey et al., *Brit. Med. J.* (1971), p. 16.

10. B. Hutchinson-Smith, *Medical Officer,* Vol. 123 (1970), p. 257.

11. Ahrens & Connor, *op. cit.*

12. D. B. Frewin et al., *Med. J. Aust.,* Vol. 2 (1978), p. 497. *See also* K. Y. Lee et al., *Lancet,* Vol. 1 (1979), p. 1110.

13. J. D. Horowitz et al., *Lancet,* Vol. 1 (1980), p. 60.

14. G. Enzi et al., *Obesity: Pathogenesis and Treatment* (New York: Academic Press, 1981).

15. B. K. Watt and A. L. Merrill, *Composition of Foods* (Washington, D.C.: USDA, 1963).

16. A. Stunkard and M. McLaren-Hume, *Arch. Intern. Med.,* Vol. 103 (1959), p. 79.

17. W. Bennett and J. Gurim, *The Dieter's Dilemma* (New York: Basic Books, 1982).

18. M. Winick, ed., *Childhood Obesity* (New York: Wiley, 1975).

19. T. Aoki, in Selvey & White, eds., *op. cit.*

20. Bennett & Gurim, *op. cit.*

21. D. Johnson and E. J. Drenick, *Arch. Intern. Med.,* Vol. 137 (1977), p. 1381.

22. Enzi et al., *op. cit.*

23. T. Gordon and W. B. Kannel, *Geriatrics,* Vol. 28 (1973), p. 80.

24. S. A. Hashim, in Enzi et al., eds, *op. cit.*

25. In Enzi et al., eds., *op. cit.*

26. Johnson & Drenick, *op. cit.*

27. S. Schachter and J. Rodin, *Obese Humans and Rats* (Potomac, Md.: Erlbaum, 1974), passim.

28. G. V. Vahonny, *Am. J. Clin. Nutr.,* Vol. 35 (1982), p. 152.

29. R. Wood, *Med. Sci. Sports,* Vol. 32 (1981).

30. L. B. Oscai and B. T. Williams, *J. Amer. Geriatr. Soc.,* Vol. 16 (1968), p. 794.

31. Bennett & Gurim, *op. cit.*

Chapter 9

1. American Heart Association, *Selected Heart Facts* (New York: 1977).
2. Ibid.
3. Ibid.
4. R. I. Levy, Address to the National Institutes of Health, November 27, 1979, mimeographed. *See also* five-year findings of hypertension detection and follow-up program summarized in *JAMA,* Vol. 242 (1979), p. 2562.
5. A. Keys, *Circulation,* Vol. 41 (1970), Supp. 1.
6. J. J. McNamara et al., *JAMA,* Vol. 216 (1971), p. 1185.
7. A. Keys, *op. cit.*
8. R. L. Holman et al., *Am. J. Pathol.,* Vol. 34 (1958), p. 209.
9. A. Keys, *op. cit.*
10. R. L. Holman, *op. cit.*
11. I. A. Prior, *Int. J. Epidem.,* Vol. 3 (1974), p. 225. *See also* I. A. Prior, *Advances in Metabolic Disorders,* Vol. 9 (1978), p. 241.
12. H. G. Mather et al., *Br. Med. J.,* Vol. 3 (1971), p. 334.
13. J. F. Kurtzke, *Epidemiology of Cerebrovascular Disease* (New York: Springer, 1969).
14. Coronary Drug Project, National Heart, Lung and Blood Institute, *JAMA,* Vol. 220 (1972), p. 996.
15. H. D. Cain et al., *Geriatrics,* Vol. 18 (1963), p. 507. *See also* M. I. Lindsay and R. E. Spiekerman, *Am. Heart J.,* Vol. 67 (1964), p. 559.
16. L. Kuller et al., *Circulation,* Vol. 24 (1966), p. 1056.
17. Levy, *op. cit.*
18. Levy, *op. cit.*
19. J. P. Henry and J. C. Cassel, *Am. J. Epidemiology,* Vol. 90 (1969), p. 171.
20. Ibid. *See also* P. H. Evans, *Lancet,* Vol. 1 (1965), p. 516.
21. Henry & Cassel, *op. cit.*
22. Ibid.
23. H. Benson, *The Relaxation Response* (New York: William Morrow, 1975).
24. M. Colgan, *New Zeal. Med. J.,* Vol. 93 (1981), p. 49.
25. Henry & Cassel, *op. cit.*
26. The Surgeon General, *The 1979 Surgeon General's Report on Smoking and Health,* DHEW, Pub. No. 017-000-0218-0 (Washington, D.C.: 1979).
27. K. Ball and R. Turner, *Lancet,* Vol. 2 (1974), p. 822.
28. W. J. McKenna et al., *Br. Heart J.,* Vol. 83 (1980), p. 493.
29. P. Astrup, *Br. Med. J.,* Vol. 4 (1972), p. 447.
30. Ibid.

31. Ball & Turner, *op. cit.*
32. Astrup, *op. cit.*
33. O. Auerbach et al., *N. Eng. J. Med.,* Vol. 273 (1965) p. 775.
34. Ball & Turner, *op. cit. See also* C. Wilhelmsson et al., *Lancet,* Vol. 1 (1975), p. 415.
35. A. Burt et al., *Lancet,* Vol. 1 (1974), p. 304.
36. S. Byers, *Am. J. Clin. Nutr.,* Vol. 6 (1958), p. 638.
37. G. V. Mann, *N. Eng. J. Med.* (1977).
38. G. Gould, *Am. J. Med.,* Vol. 11 (1951), p. 209.
39. E. H. Ahrens, *Ann. Intern. Med.,* Vol. 85 (1976), p. 87.
40. G. Slater et al. *Nutrition Reports International,* Vol. 14 (1976), p. 249. *See also* M. W. Porter et al., *Am. J. Clin. Nutr.,* Vol. 30 (1977), p. 490.
41. Coronary Drug Project, *op. cit.*
42. R. Levy, *Nutrition in the 1980's: Constraints on Our Knowledge,* eds. N. Selvey and P. L. White (New York: Alan R. Liss, 1981), p. 357.
43. R. Williams, *Nutrition Against Disease* (New York: Pitman, 1971), p. 274.
44. H. A. Kahn, *Am. J. Clin. Nutr.,* Vol. 23 (1970), p. 879.
45. C. R. Sirtoni et al., *Am. J. Clin. Nutr.,* Vol. 32 (1979), p. 1645. *See also* K. K. Carroll, *Nutr. Reviews,* Vol. 36 (1978), p. 1.
46. A. Keys and M. H. Keys, *The Benevolent Bean* (New York: Doubleday, 1967).
47. R. M. Kay and A. S. Trusswell, *Am. J. Clin. Nutr.,* Vol. 30 (1977), p. 171. *See also* M. M. Baig and J. J. Cerda, *Am. J. Clin. Nutr.,* Vol. 34 (1981), p. 50.
48. L. M. Morrison, *Geriatrics,* Vol. 13 (1958), p. 12.
49. A. Keys, *Circulation,* Vol. 41 (1970), Supp. 1. *See also* J. Stamler, *Med. Clin. North Am.,* Vol. 57 (1973), p. 5.
50. R. I. Levy and M. Feinleib, *Heart Disease,* ed. E. Braunwald (Philadelphia: W. B. Saunders, 1980), p. 1246.
51. T. Gordon et al., *Am. J. Med.,* Vol. 62 (1977), p. 707.
52. C. J. Bates et al., *Lancet,* Vol. 2 (1977), p. 611.
53. W. P. Castelli et al., *Lancet,* Vol. 2 (1977), p. 153.
54. J. J. Barboriak et al., *Alcoholism,* Vol. 3 (1979), p. 29. *See also* C. H. Hennekens et al., *JAMA,* Vol. 242 (1979), p. 1973.
55. A. Keys, *Circulation,* Vol. 41 (1970), Supp. 1.
56. R. Levy, in Selvey & White, eds. *op. cit.*
57. Ibid.
58. M. D. Haust et al., *Am. J. Pathol.,* Vol. 35 (1959), p. 265.
59. L. A. Harker et al., *Ann. N.Y. Acad. Sci.,* Vol. 275 (1976), p. 321.
60. S. Renaud and F. Lecompte, *Circ. Res.,* Vol. 27 (1970), p. 1003.
61. S. Renaud et al., in Selvey & White, eds., *op. cit.*
62. M. J. Haut and D. H. Cowan, *Am. J. Med.,* Vol. 56 (1974), p. 22.

63. A. Bordia, *Atherosclerosis* (August 1978), p. 355. *See also* D. J. Boullin, *Lancet,* Vol. 1 (1981), p. 776.

64. A. N. Makheja, *Lancet,* Vol. 1 (1979), p. 781.

65. H. Yacowitz et al., *Br. Med. J.,* Vol. 1 (1965), p. 1352.

66. S. Renaud et al., in Selvey & White, eds., *op. cit.*

67. G. W. Comstock, *Am. J. Epidemiol.,* Vol. 110 (1979), p. 375.

68. J. Yudkin, *Lancet,* Vol. 2 (1957), p. 155. *See also* J. Yudkin and J. Morland, *Am. J. Clin. Nutr.,* Vol. 20 (1967), p. 503.

69. P. T. Kus et al., *Am. J. Clin. Nutr.,* Vol. 20 (1967), p. 116.

70. G. D. Talbot, *Ann. Intern. Med.,* Vol. 54 (1961), p. 257.

71. E. D. Freis, *Circulation,* Vol. 53 (1976), p. 589.

72. National Research Council Food and Nutrition Board, *Toward Healthful Diets* (Washington, D.C.: Academy of Sciences, 1980).

73. E. D. Freis, *op. cit.*

74. R. I. Levy, *op. cit.*

75. M. E. Kosman, *JAMA,* Vol. 230 (1974), p. 5.

76. G. D. Rook et al., *Br. Heart J.,* Vol. 35 (1973), p. 87.

77. M. M. Nelson et al., *J. Nutr.,* Vol. 56 (1955), p. 49.

78. T. Kopjas, *J. Amer. Geriatr. Soc.,* Vol. 14 (1966), p. 1187.

79. L. D. Greenberg and J. F. Rinehart, *Proc. Soc. Exp. Biol. Med.,* Vol. 76 (1951), p. 580.

80. R. E. Olson, *Circulation,* Vol. 48 (1973), p. 179. *See also* R. E. Gillian et al., *Am. Heart J.,* Vol. 93 (1977), p. 444.

81. H. T. G. Williams et al., *Surg. Gynecol. Obstet.,* Vol. 132 (1971), p. 662. *See also* P. D. Livingstone and C. Jones, *Lancet,* Vol. 2 (1958), p. 602; and K. Haeger, *Vascular Diseases,* Vol. 5 (1968), p. 199.

82. A. M. Boyd et al., *Angiology,* Vol. 14 (1963), p. 198.

83. M. Steiner and J. Anastasi, *J. Clin. Invest.,* Vol. 57 (1976), p. 732.

84. J. H. Kay et al., *Surgery,* Vol. 28 (1950), p. 24. *See also* M. Zurler et al., *Ann. N.Y. Acad. Sci.,* Vol. 52 (1949), p. 180.

85. R. E. Olson, *op. cit. See also* M. K. Horwitt, *Nutr. Rev.,* Vol. 38 (1980), p. 105.

86. W. J. Hermann et al., *Am. J. Clin. Pathol.,* Vol. 72 (1979), p. 849.

87. B. Nambisan and P. A. Kurup, *Atherosclerosis,* Vol. 19 (1974), p. 191.

88. C. R. Spittle, *Lancet,* Vol. 2 (1971), p. 1278. *See also* B. Sokoloff et al., *J. Am. Geriatr. Soc.,* Vol. 14 (1966), p. 1239.

89. C. R. Spittle, *op. cit.*

90. K. J. Kingsbury et al., *Lancet,* Vol. 2 (1969).

91. M. Colgan, *Science,* Vol. 214 (1981), p. 744.

92. Chinese Academy of Medical Sciences, *Chin. Med. J.,* Vol. 92 (1979), p. 471.

93. H. A. Schroeder, *J. Chron. Dis.,* Vol. 12 (1960), p. 586. *See also* H. A.

Schroeder, *JAMA,* Vol. 95 (1966), p. 81; and M. D. Crawford et al., *Lancet,* Vol. 1 (1968), p. 827.

94. M. D. Crawford et al., *Lancet,* Vol. 3 (1971), p. 327.

95. H. A. Schroeder, *J. Chron. Dis.,* Vol. 15 (1962), p. 941. *See also* R. M. Welch and E. E. Cary, *Agric. Food Chem.,* Vol. 23 (1975), p. 479.

96. H. M. Perry et al., *Proc. 8th Annual Conference, Trace Substances in Environmental Health* (Missoula, Mont.: University of Montana, 1975), p. 51.

97. R. Riales and M. J. Albrink, *Am. J. Clin. Nutr.,* Vol. 34 (1981), p. 2670.

98. E. H. Ahrens and W. E. Connor, *Am. J. Clin. Nutr.,* Vol. 32 (1979), p. 2621.

99. D. Streja and D. Mymin, *JAMA,* Vol. 242 (1979), p. 2190.

100. R. S. Willams et al., *N. Eng. J. Med.,* Vol. 302 (1980), p. 987.

101. R. S. Paffenbarger (Paper No. 292 given at the American Heart Association Scientific Sessions, Anaheim, California, November 1979).

102. G. H. Hartung et al., *N. Eng. J. Med.,* Vol. 302 (1980), p. 357.

103. W. Erkelens et al., *JAMA,* Vol. 242 (1979), p. 2185.

104. T. Bassler, *The Marathon: Physiological, Medical, Epidemiological and Psychological Studies,* ed. P. Milvy (New York: New York Academy of Sciences, 1977), p. 579.

Chapter 10

1. American Cancer Society, "Cancer Statistics, 1982," *Ca—A Cancer Journal for Clinicians,* Vol. 32 (1982), p. 15.

2. Ibid. *See also* National Cancer Institute, *Cancer Patient Survival Reports,* No. 5 (Bethesda, Md.: 1976).

3. American Cancer Society, *op. cit.*

4. Ibid.

5. Ibid. *See also* E. Silverberg, *Ca—A Cancer Journal for Clinicians,* Ibid., p. 1.

6. R. Sutherland, *Cancer: The Significance of Delay* (London: Butterworth, 1960), passim. *See also* N. E. McKinnon, *Can. Med. Assoc. J.,* Vol. 82 (1960) p. 1308; H. Atkins, *Br. Med. J.,* Vol. 2 (1972), p. 423; and D. P. Byar, *J. Urology,* Vol. 108 (1972), p. 908.

7. The Surgeon General, *Healthy People: The Surgeon General's Report on Health Promotion and Disease Prevention.* DHEW, Pub. Nos. 79-55071 and 79-55071A (Washington, D.C.: 1979), p. 65.

8. R.V.P. Hutter, *Ca—A Cancer Journal for Clinicians,* Vol. 32 (1982), p. 2.

9. R. Doll, *Origins of Human Cancer,* Book A., eds. H. H. Hiatt et al. (Cold Spring Harbor Laboratory, 1977), p. 1. *See also* L. Pauling and E. Cameron, *Cancer and Vitamin C* (Menlo Park, Calif.: Linus Pauling Institute, 1979); and The Surgeon General *op. cit.*

10. The Surgeon General, *op. cit.* p. 104.

11. V. Saffioti, *Carcinogenic Risks: Strategies for Intervention,* eds. W. Davis and C. Rosenfeld (Lyon: WHO, International Agency for Research on Cancer, 1979).

12. The Surgeon General, *op. cit.* p. 64.

13. American Cancer Society, *op. cit.*

14. The Surgeon General, *op. cit.* p. 104. *See also* M. L. Newhouse and G. Berry, *Br. J. Indust. Med.,* Vol. 33 (1976), p. 147.

15. U.S. Dept. of Health, Education and Welfare, *HEW News,* Vol. 301, (August 29, 1975). *See also* the Food and Drug Administration, *FDA Consumer,* Vol. 10 (January 1976).

16. The Surgeon General, *op. cit.* p. 65

17. The Surgeon General, *Report on Smoking and Health,* DHEW, Pub. No. 017-000-0218-0 (Washington, D.C.: 1979).

18. American Cancer Society, *op. cit. See also* Ibid. (1981).

19. The Surgeon General, *The Health Consequences of Smoking: The Changing Cigarette,* Dept. of Health and Human Services (Washington, D.C.: 1981), passim.

20. J. L. Repace, *Bull. N.Y. Acad. Med.* (in press, 1982).

21. D. P. Rall, in Davis & Rosenfeld, *op. cit.*

22. AMA Dept. of Drugs, *AMA Drug Evaluations* 4th ed. (Littleton, Mass.: American Medical Association, 1980).

23. D. P. Rall in Davis & Rosenfeld, *op. cit. See also* AMA Dept. of Drugs, *op. cit.* passim.

24. D. Schmahl et al., *Iatrogenic Carcinogenesis* (New York: Springer-Verlag, 1977), passim.

25. M. Sun, *Science,* Vol. 214 (1981), p. 887.

26. J. W. Gofman, *Radiation and Human Health* (San Francisco: Sierra Book Club, 1981), passim.

27. R. Gibson et al., *J. Natl. Cancer Inst.,* Vol. 48 (1972), p. 301.

28. R. Mendelsohn, *Mal(e) Practice: How Doctors Manipulate Women* (New York: Contemporary Books, 1981).

29. AMA Dept. of Drugs, *op. cit.* passim.

30. Ivie G. Wayne et al., *Science,* Vol. 213 (1981), p. 909.

31. C. A. Linsell, in Davis & Rosenfeld, *op. cit.*

32. Ibid.

33. Ibid.

34. B. MacMahon, *N. Eng. J. Med.* (March 12, 1981).

35. American Cancer Society, *op. cit.*

36. Reported by the National Institutes of Health in *NIH Week* (February 6, 1982), p. 2.

37. American Cancer Society, *Cancer Prevention Study 1959–1979: A Report on Twenty Years of Progress* (New York: 1980), passim.

38. R. Weindruch and R. Walford, *Science,* Vol. 215 (1982), p. 1415.

39. K. Liu et al., *Lancet,* Vol. 2 (1979), p. 782.

40. J. Waterhouse et al., *Cancer Research,* Vol. 3. (Lyon: WHO, International Agency for Research on Cancer 1976).

41. W. Haenzel and M. Kurihara, *J. Natl. Cancer Inst.,* Vol. 40 (1964), p. 43.

42. D. P. Burkitt, *Lancet,* Vol. 2 (1972), p. 1408.

43. G. A. Glober et al., *Lancet,* Vol. 2 (1977), p. 110.

44. K. K. Carroll et al., *Can. Med. Assoc. J., Vol. 98 (1968), p. 590.*

45. J. H. Weisburger, J. Occup. Med., Vol. 18 (1976), p. 245.

46. D. Harman, *J. Gerontol.,* Vol. 26 (1971), p. 451.

47. M. L. Pearce and S. Cayton, *Lancet,* Vol. 1 (1971), p. 464.

48. F. Ederer et al., *Lancet,* Vol. 2 (1971), p. 203.

49. B. S. Mackie, *Med. J. Aust.,* Vol. 1 (1974), p. 810.

50. T. H. Maugh, *Science,* Vol. 186 (1974), p. 1198. *See also* M. B. Sporn, *Fed. Proc.,* Vol. 35 (1976), p. 1332.

51. M. B. Sporn, *Nutr. Reviews* (April 1977).

52. A. S. Evans and G. W. Comstock, *Lancet,* Vol. 2 (1981), p. 1183.

53. E. A. Rogers, *Cancer Res.,* Vol. 35 (1975), p. 2469.

54. H. F. Kraybill, *Clin. Pharmacol. Ther.,* Vol. 4 (1963), p. 73.

55. E. Cameron et al., *Cancer Res.,* Vol. 39 (1979), p. 663.

56. R. H. Yonemoto, *Int. J. Vitamin Nutr. Res.* (1979), Supp. 19.

57. J. A. Miglozzi, *Br. J. Cancer,* Vol. 35 (1977), p. 448.

58. E. Bjelke, *Scand. J. Gastroenterology,* Vol. 9 (1974), Supp. 31. *See also* E. Cameron and L. Pauling, *Cancer and Vitamin C* (Menlo Park, Calif.: Linus Pauling Institute, 1979).

59. Ibid. *See also* S. Lewin, *Vitamin C: Its Molecular Biology and Medical Potential* (London: Academic Press, 1976).

60. M. E. Shils, *Nutrition and Neoplasia* (Philadelphia: Lea & Febiger, 1973).

61. M. M. Jacobs and A. C. Griffin, *Biol. Trace Element Res.,* Vol. 1 (1979), p. 1.

62. K. A. Poirer and J. A. Milner, *Biol. Trace Element Res.,* Vol. 1 (1979), p. 25.

63. G. N. Schrauzer et al., *Bioinorganic Chem.,* Vol. 6 (1976), p. 265.

64. B. Jansson et al., *Cancer,* Vol. 36 (1975), p. 2373. *See also* R. J. Shamberger and C. E. Willis, *Clin. Lab. Sci.,* Vol. 2 (1971), p. 211.

65. R. Doll, *Origins of Human Cancer,* eds. H. H. Hiatt et al. (Cold Spring Harbor Laboratory, 1977), p. 12.

66. L. Thomas, *Daedalus,* (Winter 1977), p. 35.

Chapter 11

1. R. A. Camarini-Davalos and R. Hanover, eds., "Treatment of Early Diabetes" *Advances in Experimental Medicine and Biology,* Vol. 119. (New York: Plenum Press, 1979), passim.

2. Ibid.

3. Ibid.

4. M. E. Levin and L. Recant, *Arch. Environ. Health,* Vol. 12 (1966), p. 621. *See also* P. S. Entmacher and H. H. Marks, *Diabetes,* Vol. 14 (1965), p. 212.

5. G. M. Reaven et al., *Diabetes,* Vol. 19 (1970), p. 571. *See also* Ibid., Vol. 20 (1971), p. 416.

6. W. Oppermann et al., in Camarini-Davalos & Hanover, eds., *op. cit.* p. 177.

7. R. Luft and S. Efendic, *Acta Diabetica Lat.,* Vol. 15 (1978), p. 1.

8. C. L. Meinert et al., *Diabetes,* Vol. 19 (1970), Supp. 2, p. 789. *See also* G. L. Knatterud et al., *JAMA,* Vol. 217 (1971), p. 777.

9. T. Deckert and M. Larson, in Camarini-Davalos & Hanover, eds., *op. cit.* p. 21.

10. J. P. Felber and A. Nanotti, *Medicina Experimentalis,* Vol. 10. (1964), p. 153. *See also* G. M. Reaven et al., *J. Clin. Invest.,* Vol. 45 (1967), p. 1756.

11. J. D. Baqdade, *N. Eng. J. Med.,* Vol. 276 (1967), p. 427.

12. V. Buber, *Schweiz Med. Wschr.,* Vol. 98 (1968), p. 711.

13. J. W. Farguhar et al., *J. Clin. Invest.,* Vol. 45 (1966), p. 1648.

14. A. Antones et al., *Lancet,* Vol. 1 (1961), p. 3.

15. W. E. Conner, *Diabetes,* Vol. 12 (1963), p. 127.

16. T. A. Miettinen, *Circulation,* Vol. 44 (1971), p. 842. *See also* P. J. Nestel et al., *J. Clin. Invest.,* Vol. 48 (1969), p. 982.

17. E. A. Sims et al., *Ann. Rev. Med.,* Vol. 22 (1971), p. 235.

18. L. J. Herberg and D. L. Coleman, *Metabolism,* Vol. 26 (1977), p. 59. *See also* S. C. Woods and D. Porte, *Advances in Metabolic Disorders,* Vol. 9, eds. R. Levine and R. Luft (New York: Academic Press, 1978), p. 283; and D. Rabinowitz, *Ann. Rev. Med.,* Vol. 21 (1970), p. 241.

19. I. M. D. Jackson et al., *Lancet,* Vol. I (1969), p. 285.

20. Ibid.

21. P. A. Rudnick and K. W. Taylor, *Br. Med. J.,* Vol. 1 (1965), p. 1225. *See also* D. R. Hadden et al., *Br. Med. J.,* Vol. 3 (1975), p. 276; and J. M. Olefsky, *J. Clin Invest.,* Vol. 53 (1974), p. 64.

22. W. K. Ishmael, *Medical Times,* Vol. 94 (1966), p. 157.

23. G. D. Campbell, *South African Med. J.* (November 1963).
24. P. H. Bennett et al., *Recent Progress in Hormone Res.,* Vol. 32 (1976), p. 333.
25. National Research Council Food and Nutrition Board, *Toward Healthful Diets* (Washington, D.C.: National Academy of Sciences, 1980), p. 15.
26. G. M. Reaven, in Camarini-Davalos & Hanover, eds., *op. cit.* p. 253.
27. H. Ginsberg et al., *J. Clin. Endocrinol. Metab.,* Vol. 42 (1976), p.729. *See also* P. A. Crapo et al., *Diabetes,* Vol. 26 (1977), p. 1178.
28. G. M. Reaven, in Camarini-Davalos & Hanover, eds., *op. cit.*
29. J. R. Perkins, *Diabetologia,* Vol. 13 (1977), p. 607.
30. K. M. West, *Nutr. Rev.,* Vol. 33 (1975), p. 193.
31. T. G. Kiehm et al., *Am. J. Clin. Nutr.,* Vol. 29 (1976) p. 895. *See also* J. W. Anderson and K. Ward, *Diabetes Care,* Vol. 1 (1978), p. 77; D.J.A. Jenkins et al., *Lancet,* Vol. 2 (1977), p. 779; and G. A. Spiller and R. P. Kay, eds., *Medical Aspects of Dietary Fiber* (New York: Plenum Press, 1980), p. 175.
32. D.J.A. Jenkins, in Camarini-Davalos & Hanover, eds., *op. cit.* p. 275.
33. J. W. Anderson, *Clin. Res.,* Vol. 26 (1978), p. 719A.
34. J. W. Anderson, in Camarini-Davalos & Hanover, eds., *op. cit.* p. 263.
35. G. M. Reaven, in Camarini-Davalos & Hanover, eds., *op. cit.*
36. Ibid.
37. H. E. Axelrod, *Am. J. Physiol.,* Vol. 165 (1951), p. 604.
38. A. S. Reddi et al., in Camarini-Davalos & Hanover, eds., *op. cit.* p. 243.
39. P. D. Livingstone and C. Jones, *Lancet,* Vol. 2 (1958), p. 602. *See also* K. Haeger, *Vascular Diseases,* Vol. 5 (1968), p. 199.
40. W. J. Hermann et al., *Am. J. Clin. Pathol.,* Vol. 72 (1979), p. 849.
41. G. J. Mann, *Perspectives in Biology and Medicine* (Winter 1974).
42. R. M. Gould, *Brain Res.,* Vol. 117 (1976), p. 168.
43. D. A. Greene, et al., *J. Clin. Invest.,* Vol. 55 (1975), p. 1326.
44. J. D. Ward et al., *Lancet,* Vol. 1 (1971), p. 428.
45. R. S. Clements, in Camarini-Davalos & Hanover, eds., *op. cit.* p. 287.
46. R. A. Camarini-Davalos and S. S. Fayans in Camarini-Davalos & Hanover, eds., *op. cit.* pp. 1 and 7.
47. G. J. Everson and R. E. Shrader, *J. Nutr.,* Vol. 94 (1968), p. 89.
48. W. Mertz, *Proc. Nutr. Soc.,* Vol. 33 (1974), p. 307.
49. W. Mertz et al., *J. Nutr.,* Vol. 86 (1965), p. 107.
50. W. H. Glinsmann and W. Mertz, *Metab. Clin. Exp.,* Vol. 15 (1966), p. 510. *See also* L. L. Hopkins and M. G. Price, *Proc. West. Hemisphere Nutr. Cong. II,* Vol. 2, American Medical Association (Acton, Mass.: Publishing Sciences Group, 1968), p. 40.

51. R. Riales and M. Albrink, *Am. J. Clin. Nutr.* Vol. 34 (1981), p. 2670.
52. S. Calstrom et al., *Lancet,* Vol. 1 (1964), p. 331.
53. N. B. Ruderman et al., *Diabetes,* Vol. 28 (1979), Supp. 1, p. 29.
54. D. Streja and D. Mymin, *JAMA,* Vol. 242 (1979), p. 2190.
55. R. Coce et al., in Camarino-Davalos & Hanover, eds., *op. cit.* p. 453.

Chapter 12

1. Environmental Protection Agency, Water Supply Division, Washington, D.C., personal communications, March 1982.
2. M. Sun, *Science,* Vol. 216 (1982), p. 275.
3. EPA, *op. cit.*
4. J. E. Brody, *Jane Brody's Nutrition Book* (New York: W. W. Norton, 1981), p. 468.
5. AMA Dept. of Drugs, *AMA Drug Evaluations,* 4th ed. (Littleton, Mass.: American Medical Association, 1980), p. 678. *See also* J. Bichler, *DES Daughter* (New York: Avon, 1981).
6. G. L. Waldbott, *Health Effects of Environment Pollutants* (St. Louis: Mosby, 1973).
7. A. Tappel, *Micronutrient Interactions: Vitamins, Minerals and Hazardous Elements,* eds. O. A. Levander and L. Cheng. *Ann. N.Y. Acad. Sci.,* Vol. 355 (New York: New York Academy of Sciences, 1980).
8. J. M. Cleveland and T. F. Rees, *Science,* Vol. 212 (1981), p. 1506.
9. National Academy of Science, *Lead: Airborne Lead in Perspective* (Washington, D.C., 1972).
10. H. Needleman et al., *N. Eng. J. Med.,* Vol. 300 (1979), p. 689. *See also* H. Waldron and D. Stofen, *Subclinical Lead Poisoning* (New York: Academic Press, 1974).
11. D. G. Mitchell and K. M. Aldous, *Environ. Health Perspect.,* Vol. 7 (1974), p. 59.
12. P. J. Barlow and M. Kapel, *Hair, Trace Elements and Human Illness,* eds. A. C. Brown and R. G. Crounse (New York: Praeger, 1980). *See also* R. O. Pihl and M. Parkes, *Science,* Vol. 198 (1977), p. 204.
13. J. Bjorksten, *Longevity—A Quest* (Madison, Wisc.: Bjorksten Research Foundation, 1981).
14. N. Childers and G. M. Russo, *Childers' Diet to Stop Arthritis* (prepublication copy, 1981).
15. F. R. Senti, *Nutrients in Processed Foods,* ed. American Medical Association Council on Foods and Nutrition (Acton Mass.: Publishing Sciences Group, 1974).
16. M. Berenboum, *Science,* Vol. 201 (1978), p. 532.
17. M. Ashwood Smith et al., *Nature* (London), Vol. 285 (1980), p. 407

18. F. R. Senti, in AMA Council on Foods and Nutrition, ed., *op. cit.*
19. T. W. Anderson, *Lancet,* Vol. 2 (1973), p. 298.
20. B. Thafvelin, *Nature* (London), Vol. 186 (1960), p. 1169.
21. C. Holden, *Science,* Vol. 214 (1981).
22. Editorial, *Science,* Vol. 180 (1973), p. 1038. *See also* N. Wade, *Science,* Vol. 179 (1973), p. 775.
23. The Surgeon General, *Healthy People: The Surgeon General's Report on Health Promotion and Disease Prevention,* DHEW, Pub. Nos. 79-55071 and 79-55071A (Washington, D.C.: 1979).
24. H. N. Beaty and R. G. Petersdorf, *Ann. Int. Med.,* Vol. 65 (1966), p. 641.
25. G. Gerbner et al., *N. Eng. J. Med.,* Vol. 305 (1981), p. 901.

Appendix 1

1. V. Herbert, *Nutrition Cultism* (Philadelphia: Stickley, 1980), passim.
2. R. J. Williams, *Nutrition Against Disease* (New York: Bantam Books, 1978), passim.
3. A. Keys, *Nutrition in the 1980's: Constraints on Our Knowledge,* eds. N. Selvey and P. L. White (New York: Alan R. Liss, 1981), p. 35.
4. Consumer Reports editors, *The Medicine Show,* 5th ed. (New York: Pantheon, 1980).
5. N. Wade, *Science,* Vol. 180 (1973), p. 1038.
6. Ibid.
7. B. Rosenthal et al., *The Progressive* (November 1976).
8. *Report of the White House Conference on Food, Nutrition and Health 1969* (Washington, D. C.: USGPO, 1970).
9. N. Wade, *Science,* Vol. 179 (1973), p. 776.
10. AMA Dept. of Drugs, *AMA Drug Evaluations,* 4th ed. (Littleton, Mass.: American Medical Association, 1980), passim.

INDEX